Electro-Homoeopathic Medicine

A New Medical System

Being

A Popular and Domestic Guide Founded on Experience

By

Count Cesar Mattei

Translated By
R M Theobald

Second Editon

Originals
Delhi

Second Edition Published 1891

Reprinted with New Introduction 2017

Count Cesare Mattei (1809–1896)

ISBN 13: 978-81-8454-172-4
ISBN 10: 81-8454-172-4

Published By
Originals
A-6, Second Floor, Nimri Commercial Centre,
Ashok Vihar Phase-4, Delhi - 110 052 (India)
Tei.: +91 11 2730 2453 Fax: 011 4706 1936
website: www.Lppindia.com
e-mail: info@Lppindia.com

Printed At
D K Fine Art Press P Ltd.
Delhi-110052

PRINTED IN INDIA

Prof. Dr. Debasish Kundu

M.D.H., F.F.Hom, F.I.H.M.S., Ph.D.(U.S.A.), D.Sc.(Colombo)

Fellow of International Holistic Medical Society, CA, U.S.A.

Fellow of Foundation of Homeopathy, NY, U.S.A.

Fellow of World E. Homeopathy System of Medical Council, Hong Kong,

Faculty, International Holistic Medical Society,CA, U.S.A.,

Vice-President, American Nutritional Medical Association, CA, U.S.A.

Visiting Professor, Khulna Homeopathic Medical College & Hospital, Khulna, Bangladesh

Former Director General, Mooreland University, U.S.A.

Author:

Materia Medica for the New Age Man,

Materia Medica and Practice of Medicine in Electro Homeopathy,

Pharmacodynamics in Spagyric Medicine,

Diseases of Women,

Natural Medicines,

A Clinical Treatise on Cancer,

Aids & Your Sex Life,

Aids & Homeopathy,

Essentials of Acupuncture, etc.

Recipient, Royal Assyrian Order of Merit,

Laureate, Dag Hammarskjold Award for Medicine,

Editor In Chief, International Journal of Homeopathy & Natural Medicines, Science PG, U.S.A.

Editor in Chief, The Internet Journal of Herbal and Plant Medicine, U.S.A.

Introduction

Count Cesare Mattei 1809 – 1896, a slightly unhinged, self-taught medicine man and politician who had developed his own system of healing that he said harnessed the life energy (electricity) of plants to heal all of Man's ills, called Electro Homoeopathy, which is widely enjoyed today as Spagyric medicine. "Electrohomoeopathy", a method he invented and believed in strongly as a powerful curative practice, which combined the use of herbs with electric bio-energy from plants and homoeopathy.

The principles of electro-homoeopathy, a new science was published by Count Cesar Mattei, of Bologna in 1874 in Italian language which was then published in other languages. It includes a catalogue of diseases cured by electro-homoeopathy with the indication of the remedies of curing them.

It has been translated in English by R M Theobald and was published in 1888 by David Stott of 370 Oxford Street W, London.

Mattei's Electro Homoeopathy has been brought to India by Dr H D Banerjee, who established first Electro Homoeopathy medical college in Calcutta in 1909 which is relevant from the correspondence between Dr Banerjee and Maria Ventrouli Mattei. According to M V Mattei, after the demise of Cesare Mattei, Electro Homoeopathy has been divided into several schools, Krauss, Muller, Sauter, Ponzio, Zimpel and so on, but according to the version of the adopted son of Count Mattei these were just imitations and 'were emerged after the death of Count Mattei, just as Minerva came out armed from the head of Jupiter' (see the Foreword of Dr H D Banerjee's Lectures on Materia Medica by M V Mattei, dated 18 June, 1909).

This is the masterpiece from the great master, let's begin the journey into the galaxy of true Mattei philosophy.

ELECTRO-HOMŒOPATHIC MEDICINE.

ELECTRO-HOMŒOPATHIC MEDICINE

A NEW MEDICAL SYSTEM

BEING

A POPULAR AND DOMESTIC GUIDE FOUNDED ON EXPERIENCE

BY

COUNT CESAR MATTEI

TRANSLATED BY

R. M. THEOBALD, M.A., M.R.C.S.

SECOND EDITION.

LONDON
DAVID STOTT, 370, OXFORD STREET, W.
MDCCCXCI

TO FRIENDS OF ELECTRO-HOMŒOPATHY.

I HAVE abstained until now from publishing a book explaining the theory of Electro-Homœopathy, wishing to establish the new therapeusis by repeated experiences; which will explain why I have always limited myself to those fundamental facts which are indispensable to those who wish to prove by actual experiment the efficacy of my remedies.

After twenty-five years of trial, which have led to successful results, I can now offer the fruits or my studies and the results of my experience. It remains for my friends to take it up and spread it through the world, as something which belongs to you personally.

COMTE CÉSAR MATTEI.

TRANSLATOR'S PREFACE TO THE FIRST EDITION.

Having been accustomed now for nine years to the very frequent use of the Electro-Homœopathic remedies introduced by Count Mattei, it has appeared desirable that the principles, aims, methods, and professions of this system should be represented in a more complete and authoritative manner than that of the small handbooks of treatment, which are all that have been hitherto accessible to the British public. The following pages contain Count Mattei's latest and most matured exposition of Electro-Homœopathy, and as such I commend it to the candid examination of both professional and lay readers.

Those who have carefully experimented with Electro-Homœopathic remedies know that they are capable of exercising extraordinary therapeutic action in many cases which are not amenable to any other known treatment. So far as the relation of these remedies to ordinary Homœopathy is concerned, I regard them myself as homœopathic remedies of very large range of action, the most polychræstic of the polychræsts; so much so, that they may be applied to constitutional types, according to the indications specified by the discoverer. Neither the Count nor any of his genuine disciples are disposed to undervalue the transcendent merit of Hahnemann, as the greatest medical explorer and the profoundest medical philosopher that the world has yet seen. Electro-Homœopathy is an extension and simplification of Hahnemannian homœopathy. Those who have endeavoured faithfully to apply ordinary homœopathy according to the directions of Hahnemann, know how prodigiously difficult it is to find a clue to the perplexities of the *Materia Medica*, so as to bring its resources within the grasp of persons endowed with an ordinary measure of working capacity, and a limited time for attention to individual cases.

The real difficulty with homœopathy is not in the theory—which is as well demonstrated as any other ascertained law of nature—but in the practice. It seems almost beyond the reach of human faculties to wield such a mighty mass of isolated facts, and bring them into actual application. It is too ideal: its administration requires a *corps* of heaven-born *illuminati*, endowed with an insight or an inspiration not granted to ordinary mortals. It is too esoteric; it postulates a higher order of faculties than that of normal human development. That it will be simplified, as it is more diligently worked, I have not the shadow of a doubt; the method of "key-notes" is a great advance in this direction. Meanwhile, Electro-Homœopathy presents itself as a system in which the rigid individualization of homœopathy is not required; the most important requisites being a careful study of the few constitutional types which characterize the individuals of the human family.

My first experiment with Count Mattei's remedies was many years ago, in the case of a young lady, reduced to the last extremity of exhaustion and emaciation by marasmus or wasting disease of the intestines. Ordinary homœopathic treatment by myself and those who studied the case in consultation with me produced only unimportant mitigation of symptoms; and in sheer despair I fell back upon Electro-Homœopathy. Under the use of Scrofoloso and other remedies she rapidly recovered; she regained her lost plumpness; she is now married, and the healthy, happy mother of a family. Other cases, not less striking, have repeatedly occurred. The magical and marvellous operation of these remedies is a perpetual surprise even to those who have long used them. And the simplicity of their administration brings the healing art within reach of all who care to devote to it a moderate amount of thought, study, and observation.

It is important, however, to observe that there is no real rivalry between Electro and ordinary Homœopathy. No one, who has witnessed the "safe, swift, and sweet" efficacy of a well-selected Homœopathic remedy, can consent to forego the advantages of such potent remedial agencies. Nor does Count Mattei desire this. He claims for his system that the remedies are illustrative in a conspicuous degree of the homœopathic law; and for my part I would not allow Anti-scrofoloso or Anticanceroso to eject Sulphur and Calcarea any more than I would permit volunteers to be ejected by the regular army, or the navy by the militia. All true specifics form a holy alliance in the great warfare with suffering and disease; and although the sphere of action of various remedies may seem to overlap, yet this is an indication that science is immature, rather than that nature is confused.

In concluding these brief introductory remarks I would call attention to the interesting letter—which I retain in its original French garb—in which the Count authorizes my translation.

R. M. Theobald.

5, Grosvenor Street, W.,
August, 1888.

AUTHOR'S PREFACE TO THE ENGLISH TRANSLATION.

À MONSIEUR LE DOCTEUR THÉOBALD.

ROCHETTA, 15 *Oct.*, 1887.

MON CHER DOCTEUR,

Il y a quelque temps que de l'Angleterre et des pays ou l'on parle la langue de Shakespeare on m'écrit pour me faire connaître la nécessité de traduire en Anglais mon livre, " Médecine Electroméopatique, ou Nouvelle Thérapeutique Expérimentale."

Persuadé enfin que c'est le désir de la plupart de mes amis de voir paraître cette traduction, c'est à vous, Monsieur le Docteur, que j'accorde l'autorisation de la faire.

Comme ce livre de Médecine à été imprimé en 1883, et vous savez qu' après ce temps là j'ai découvert de nouveaux remèdes, qu' on trouve indiqués dans mes brochures postérieures (Anti-scrofoloso Giappone, Dom-Fin, Marina et Lord) il est nécessaire à présent qu'ils soient mis à leur place dans le corps de cette traduction.

Mais une modification très importante que j'ai

apportée dans mon Vade Mecum 7e edition, aux règles de l'application des Electricités, d' après la découverte des Drs. Chazarin et Dècle sur les lois de la polarité humaine, mérite bien toute votre attention, et je vous prie, Cher Docteur, de vouloir traiter cette partie comme son importance l'exige.

Agréez l'expression de ma gratitude.

Votre,

MATTEI.

PREFACE TO THE SECOND EDITION.

The very favourable reception which has been given by the English public all over the world to this translation of Count Mattei's latest and most matured exposition of his system of Electro-Homœopathy would have led to an earlier issue of this Second Edition, were it not that the publication has been delayed by the necessity of making arrangements for the right of continuous re-publication in the future.

The subject of Electro-Homœopathy, and its special claim on public notice, has been fully brought before the public by the papers written in various periodicals, especially Lady Paget's article in *The National Review* and Mr. Stead's very admirable historic and biographic surveys of the system in *The Review of Reviews*. It is now pretty generally allowed that the system of Count Mattei has vindicated its claim to earnest and practical investigation. Testimonies to its value are constantly accumulating, and its representatives may now be found in civilized countries all over the world.

My own conviction regarding them is that they

form a large and important province of the older Homœopathy of Hahnemann, and that the two are destined to work side by side in friendly co-operation. And so far as Electro-Homœopathy is approved, its success is a witness in favour of the more refined, infinitesimal Homœopathy of the earlier Hahnemannians rather than the somewhat coarse material methods of allopathizing with Homœopathic resources, which in many places have supplanted it. The globules of Mattei, and his first, second, third, and even higher dilutions, help to authenticate the claim made by the best practitioners of Homœopathy that medicine should be administered in such a form that its mere physical, chemical, and physiological qualities retreat into the invisible, imponderable, insensible conditions of infinitesimal substances. Here chemical analysis can have no place: we do not pretend to employ such measures and weights as even the most delicate scales and meters of the laboratory can verify. And therefore, when the analyst reports that he can only find sugar or water or spirit in our preparations, we have only to thank him for confirming the sincerity of our infinitesimal professions. We accept his analysis, while we demur to his assumption that all the potencies of matter are capable of detection by the tests and re-agents which he employs. It is necessary to make this principle well understood, because some of our friends have been painfully surprised and embarrassed by the confident assertions of competent chemists that our agents are destitute of remedial force, simply because they find nothing which can be registered in a formula or expressed by decimals. It seldom occurs to our scandalized friends to consider that some of the most virulent poisons in nature—poisons of plants, poisons of serpents, poisons of atmospheres—would yield equally negative results in the same investigation. The truth is that the ruling medical faculty has surrendered itself to the viceroyalty of chemists and microscopists—a microbe must be found for every disease and a chemic symbol for every remedy; and so the whole realm of infinitesimal and occult forces is entirely withdrawn from its observation. We, however, owe no allegiance to the Bureau of the Chemical Department of the Scientific State, and we decline to dress in their livery.

So far as Electro-Homœopathy is concerned, it is necessary that we should stoutly vindicate its claim to be judged by vital, and not mechanical, tests. And it may here be added that the limits of desirable, or even necessary, attenuation are by no means defined by the directions given in the text of this volume. Those who are making practical use of our methods will do well to remember that its best results have often been achieved by the most refined use of the medicines, and that while in most cases the first dilution is not too strong, in a large number of deeply-rooted chronic disorders relief or cure must be sought by the use of second, or even third, "glasses," or dilutions; and often, even while these are employed, the dose must not be too frequent. These are practical matters which can scarcely be expressed in definite rules; experience must determine in each case what degree of attenuation should be employed.

It would have been possible to expand this already somewhat too ample volume, by including a number of diseases which are not directly mentioned. But inasmuch as in all diseases treated by Electro-Homœopathy the first consideration in the selection of remedies is the type to which the patient belongs, so the treatment of cases not directly described may in all cases be inferred by a study of the general law of selection, and their application to analogous cases. It is indeed in this that the special advantage of Electro-Homœopathy consists. It does not profess to individualize the case, as in the delicate medical portraiture of ordinary Homœopathy. It is enabled by the singularly comprehensive range of action of the remedies it employs to treat cases according to their constitutional type, while the peculiarities of the individual case are utilized in deciding the potency and combinations of the medicines. In all cases the clue to a prescription must be sought for, not only in the special rubric of the case, but in the chapter which treats on general Indications, and the description of the sphere of action of the remedies.

A preface is not the place for recording detailed cases; but I may be permitted to refer to some which have come under my own care and observation, illustrating the action of the several groups of remedies which Electro-Homœopathy employs.

First as to the *Angioitic* group: In heart diseases the efficacy of these is undoubted. A short time since I saw a child suffering from Pericarditis, breathless, unable to lie, emaciated, pallid, suffering with the pain and anguish peculiar to heart disease. In a few days all these symptoms subsided, and the child, without losing all traces of heart disease, ceased to be inconvenienced by it. In other cases the heart murmur, showing valvular disease, has gradually ceased.

In *Scrofoloso*, remedies with their wide range of action have been useful; for instance, in an inveterate case of Eczema of twenty years' continuance; in another of Acne, with pustular eruption over a large part of the body; Cataract in another case; in innumerable cases of Dyspepsia of various types; in Rheumatism, in its chronic form, with extreme sensitiveness to atmospheric changes; and in many inveterate Neuralgias.

The *Canceroso* remedies generally succeed in arresting the advance of Cancer. Even in inveterate cases, where cure is impossible, symptoms are so mitigated that the worst, most painful, most offensive features of the disease are reduced to minimum. In one case the large cancerous mass was completely separated, and a fair degree of health restored. In many cases the disease has ceased to be active and the patient almost able to ignore it. A short time since I had occasion to treat a most remarkable case of tumour of the eye—the eyeball projecting beyond the orbit, raised on the top of the morbid mass, giving a most extraordinary appearance to the face, as if the eye belonged to the tumour, not to the patient—a hideous caricature of a human face. This case was so wonderfully benefited as to astonish all the neighbourhood, and bring the Electro remedies into very great favour.

In all these cases the corresponding electricities have been generally used. These external remedies—though often used internally also—are important aids to treatment, and that not only in relieving pain, but in subduing disease and assisting in the absorption and resolution of the morbid products of organic disease.

In the fervent hope that the light of this book may be a faithful guide to many in the treatment of inveterate and painful disease, this Second Edition is now launched into circulation.

R. M. Theobald.

5, Grosvenor Street, W.,
April, 1891.

TABLE OF CONTENTS.

INTRODUCTION.

THE human body is composed of blood and lymph, two substances to which is entrusted the constant nutrition and preservation of the different parts of the organism, which, though different in themselves, both in form and in the functions they are called upon to discharge, are, notwithstanding, essentially similar, since they are all primarily composed of blood and lymph, and perpetually receive their nutrition from these two elements.

Any change in one or the other of these liquids must necessarily lead to a change in the normal state of the individual, and produce an abnormal or pathologic state. In accepting this fundamental theory, as simple as it is true, it is easy to understand that the composition of my remedies, called *electro-homœopathic* on account of their instant and efficacious action, must embrace a number of simple medicinal principles, which, in virtue of their nature and their mode of action on the whole body and on the different parts of which it is composed, must respond to the combined requirements of the various morbid elements, which, by changing the normal state of the blood and the lymph, create all varieties of disease—that is to say, all those hostile elements which oppose themselves to the free exercise of our organic functions.

We are indebted to the great Hahnemann for the discovery of the *specific nature of remedies.*

Still, Hahnemann's doctrine, being founded on the use of single remedies, limits itself to fighting against symptoms; in following his system, only one medicine is given at a time, and it is on this important point that I part company with him.

If I allow with him that a single remedy is capable of a simple action bearing only on one point, yet I do not admit that this action can antidote the cause of most diseases which are generally complicated. On the other hand, I can affirm that the complex remedies which constitute the electro-homœopathic materia medica, combat and destroy disease in its primary origin, so that, treated according to this specific method, no relapse need be feared, no return in altered form is possible.

I do not conceal from myself the fact that this assertion may appear hazardous to some of my readers. Nevertheless, contrary to all that has hitherto been realized in the field of medicine, I have allowed my theory to await the test of experience, and as this experience has been crowned by undoubted success, and by cures which have been continuously effected in all classes of society, during the space of twenty-five years, I can unhesitatingly affirm that my complex remedies, that is to say, my electro-homœopathic system of medicine, is the only true and efficient healing force, since it destroys the very germs of disease in the organism, by purifying the vital fluids in which they circulate and grow.

It is therefore evident that Hahnemann's system is far from having spoken its last word, and that if the honour of having laid the unalterable basis of a new materia medica must be given to him, he has not completely reduced it to practice.

In fact, every work of nature is constituted by the fusion of different simple elements; and it is on this principle, which has its own application in every separate case, that I have founded my system. It is, in my opinion, indispensable to bring several medicines into combined action and co-operation, which, harmoniously united, constitute a potent leverage capable of overcoming every obstacle which resists the restoration of the organism to health and soundness.

For me this unity of therapeutic action is a composite made up of many parts, which, blending in united action, constitute a veritable unity; it is a harmonious co-operation towards one result, the aim of which is complete cure. Consequently the unity of remedies which is now practised by the homœopaths is a radical mistake, which has much retarded the real progress of homœopathic science.

Experience has convinced me that, in order to cure a disease which consists of a great number of symptoms, the combined action of several remedies is required by which the various manifestations of the morbid principle in the different parts of the organism which are attacked, may be successfully combated. Whilst the homœopathic method, as practised by Hahnemann, only admits a single remedy at a time in the treatment of disease, and accordingly aims in the action of its remedies at one description of tissue at a time, or one definite point which may or may not be the tissue or the part which is most seriously affected, still the other tissues, which are also attacked, are only indirectly acted on by a kind of reflected force, or else they remain entirely unaffected.

If this is the case, such a cure must be regarded as incomplete; for even if the actual disease has been overcome by the single remedy, yet the morbid principle itself has not been removed or destroyed; it still remains and manifests itself by secondary symptoms whenever the general health is affected. It is undoubtedly true that in every special case the remedies are changed, according to the law which guides practice, whenever new symptoms present themselves; but it is no less true, that if during the short period during which an acute disease lasts the medicine is changed at every new phase, there is danger lest the effectual potency of each may be lost while one follows another in such rapid succession that the only result may be an aggravation in the state of the patient. If, however, the origin itself is attacked by the complex remedies of electro-homœopathy, which fasten upon it in each one of its symptoms, the disease can no longer develop, its cause being removed. It is not even necessary that all the possible symptoms should have appeared, since while combating those which are most conspicuous, those which are secondary and subordinate are anticipated and their development arrested.

My electro-homœopathic remedies therefore constitute a great advance in the homœopathic field. I know well the determined opposition with which they are confronted by the medical schools; but in spite of all obstacles, I persevere for the sake of suffering humanity.

By my electro-homœopathic system I have endeavoured to put within reach of the disordered blood and lymph the substance most fitted to cure them, and to rescue each special organ from the hostile forces which prevent the free exercise of its functions, without doing violence to it by the use of remedies which have no power of effecting a radical cure. Here, in few words, is my theory, and my complex or electro-homœopathic remedies have no other import. For each affection of the organism, whether general or local, affecting one organ or a group of organs, there are remedies, which by their complexity cover not simply the majority of the symptoms, but the totality of them, so that the simultaneous action of these different medicines removes at once the cause and the effects.

Moreover, it is easily seen that my electro-homœopathy, which introduces such a great reform in the homœopathic therapeutics of Hahnemann, rests also on that physiological law which controls the sympathy and attraction under which all the functions of animal and vegetable life are carried on—a law of selection, of assimilation, of relation, by which useful substances are appropriated and absorbed, while substances which are useless or which are alien are rejected.

The organism itself makes this selection in a group of attenuated and potentized remedies; it chooses that which is required for its cure.

Thus, given a compound remedy, certain of its elements will only be utilized by the diseased organism when it finds in it a morbid state, or in the disease itself something to which it is naturally antagonistic. The other elements of the same remedy must necessarily be completely useless—that is to say, they have no medical action either good or bad. Only on this principle can we explain how it is that a simple or composite remedy, although it may be homœopathically related to some forms of disease, is entirely ignored by an entirely healthy organism; and evidently such a law is not applicable when the doses are no longer such as homœopathy employs, but take the massive proportions of allopathic medication,—doses, that is to say, which are measurable and ponderable.

Each specific is formed, as I have already said, of several medicines, which in their combination completely cover and control the group of organs which they are intended to act upon. Now in the complexity of these remedies there are some which pass directly into the mass of the blood, and here all the medicines which each specific includes being brought into relation with suffering organs, unite their action, the primary disease being in exact correspondence with the specific which is administered.

In fact, the organ which is affected absorbs the medicines which are appropriate to it: the other medicines, being attenuated, are in their turn absorbed by other tissues and other organs. Now, if before an organ is completely restored, or while it is disordered, another organ is attacked, in spite of the complexity of the remedies we must have recourse to those which are specifically adapted to combat the morbid condition of the organ last attacked, alternating the two specifics according to this reason of the case.

In fine, I affirm that homœopathy, using simple agents, whose action is symptomatic and limited, will remain a system of palliative treatment, not curative, by isolated remedies; while my process of treatment has two entirely distinct forms of action: one of these, purely organic, only felt by the organs which are primarily or secondarily attacked, but very comprehensive owing to the complex nature of the remedy; the other, a constitutional action, confronting the essential cause of the malady which it antidotes. This action may be utilized even during a condition of health, in the case of the scrofoloso medicines, since the cause of every disease may exist in a latent form before any purely external manifestation of its presence has taken place.

The importance of such a medical system is still more obvious if we consider that just as a healthy organism requires a variety of nutritive principles to maintain the balance of health, so also a diseased organism must appropriate to itself not one only, but many therapeutic agents. Electro-homœopathy, therefore, is nothing else than a sort of restorative nutrition, given under the form of medicine.

I can affirm that, thanks to continuous and repeated cures during more than twenty-five years, I have succeeded in discovering a combination of these remedies which may be considered perfect; a discovery which entitles me to repeat that the new application of my theory of homœopathy is definitely and beneficially assured. In fact, one of my specifics possesses not only a direct action on the mass of the blood or the lymph, but a special action on one or many organs or tissues, and on all the parts which are dependent upon them. For such is the multiplicity of symptoms in any disease of a special organ, that a disturbing influence is communicated to all the organs or tissues that depend upon it. If then, with a single remedy, we can often bring about a very rapid cure of acute diseases, one can readily imagine the success which can be secured by my specifics, which are complex remedies, and which I have called, on account of the rapidity of their action, electro-homœopathic. I assert, also, that in the same individual one single remedy may succeed in curing several organs; for the potentized remedies have a real action on the organism which is exerted as often as the condition of the organism demands it.

A remedy which can cure separately an acute affection of the lungs, or of the heart, or of the intestines, will be similarly effectual in a chronic case where all these organs are simultaneously affected.

Accordingly, when a disease has to be treated, whether acute or chronic, instead of attacking it by a single remedy—that is, at one point—we can, with my electro-homœopathic or complex specifics, cover all the various symptoms of the disease. Those organs which are less seriously affected will receive a proportionate degree of relief; thus the disease will be compassed by one single specific, although it may be necessary in the course of treatment to alternate this with other specifics, in order to meet symptoms as they arise, until the totality of them has disappeared.

It is easy to see how impossible it is to select with invariable precision the single remedy which a chronic state requires; it is indeed impossible, unless the selection is favoured by chance. With my specifics, on the contrary, we have, even before making use of them, a certainty that they will be effectual; provided there is still any vital force left we may be sure of relief; and if the organs are not profoundly affected, we may rely with certainty on a cure.

And even in such acute cases as do not involve very great constitutional disturbance, and where a single remedy might be sufficient to effect a cure, my electro-homœopathic remedies show themselves still superior to this single remedy; and, above all, the application of my specifics is so simple that, provided the diagnosis has given a thoroughly accurate idea of the cause of the disease (it does not much matter how this is ascertained), they always act in a complete and decisive way.

In fact, if one organ only is attacked, the electro-homœopathic specific will cure it better than any other remedy, since it will infallibly supply to all the tissues of the affected organs the substances which are essential to their cure, whatever the particular symptoms may be. I can even affirm that in this case the cure will be radical, because the curative agent will pervade the whole organism, working at one and the same time on the morbid state itself, and on all that is derived from it.

The practice of homœopaths is to indicate the method of using their remedies by such directions as the following: Dropsy, such a remedy; Convulsions, such a remedy. It is not thus that we must proceed. For convulsions may arise from many different causes. If, for example, they are produced by worms, they cannot be met by a remedy which cures the impurity of the blood, and *vice versâ*. One single remedy is not sufficient for dropsy; the remedy which cures ascites is by no means suitable for hydro-pericarditis, or ovarian disease. But in each of these cases we must make use of the remedies which have a special affinity for the organ which is the source of the effusion.

In the composition of my specifics I have found it necessary to take into consideration the sympathetic relations that must exist, not only between those different medicines which enter into the formation of a single specific, and which are adapted to act in harmony with one another; but I have also been forced to consider the relations between these medicines and those which enter into the formation of other specifics—thus securing the efficiency of all combinations. For as all, or several of these specifics, may be required to act together, it was necessary to provide that no one substance entering into the composition of one of them should be liable to counteract the action of any of the others.

Thus the various specifics must be united together by a harmonious relation identical with that which binds together the different substances which enter into the composition of any one. No antagonism must be suffered to exist among them, no liability for one to be absorbed into another; for if one and the same specific should contain two medicines possessing the same qualities, and having the same action, the remedies would lose their complex character, and their separate action would be destroyed.

It is therefore necessary to know how to group in a precise and rational way those remedies which are best adapted to combat the diseases which their specific powers are required to meet, so that we may be perfectly sure that the specific power is fully attained.

It now remains only that I should explain how it is not necessary, in using my specific medicines, to suspend their curative action in order that the reaction between disease and medicine may be operative. This persistent curative action I affirm, without intending entirely to deny the theory formulated by Hahnemann as to the reaction which arises when the organ is saturated by one medicinal agent, so as to completely lose the power, often for considerable space of time, of being influenced by other remedies—without, I repeat, wishing to deny such a reaction, the reality of which is, indeed, demonstrated by extraordinary cases arising in persons of exceptionally sensitive temperament, I will only remark that those who administer homœopathic medicines are often wrong in giving one single remedy whose action is very prolonged. Practice of this order is scarcely possible except for such a genius as Hahnemann, who, with vast and cultivated intelligence, and profound acquaintance with the primary action of drugs, united a subtlety of intuition which enabled him to select his remedies with almost unerring precision.

But how can a conscientious physician who does not possess this illumination, this power of instantaneous discernment which was Hahnemann's almost unique gift—how can a practitioner less magnificently endowed select a remedy, and wait in a state of masterly inactivity twenty, thirty, and even forty days' till the reaction comes? Can he thus wait without hesitation, with no tremor of misgiving while the disease is advancing from day to day? And where shall we find the patient who possesses such confidence in the efficiency of the selected medicine as to be able thus to wait patiently and confidently the result of such a protracted experiment?

If, then, this theory of reaction has in it an element of truth, it is practically an illusion, since, I once more affirm, this power of undergoing a favourable reaction after so long intervals is a peculiarity of exceptional organisms; and even if we can calculate on such a marvellous result, it is only when we can be sure that the remedy has been chosen with perfect accuracy. For if it does not cover all the characteristic symptoms its action becomes almost null, and in the majority of cases it is futile to make another twenty days' experiment after the first has proved abortive.

On the other hand, with my electro-homœopathic system it is not necessary to wait for this far-off reaction: the medicines have, all of them, a definite aim, an immediate action; they can never produce any serious aggravation; no reaction or crisis is necessary, consequently there is no need to suspend the action of the remedy.

Indeed, every organ which is sufficiently saturated with its specific will cease to absorb it; but the beneficial action will then be passed on to other organs, more recently attacked, which will continue to assimilate the substances which they require, and the cure of one will facilitate that of another, or even a partial amendment in one organ may prepare the way for the perfect cure of another.

Consider the fact that plants are always exposed to the action of air, of earth and of heat, and yet leaves and flowers only appear and grow at one season—the springing time of their life. Even so we all have the blood which circulates in the veins and gives life, and yet after a certain age our growth is arrested, and at certain seasons of the year our bodies undergo modifications peculiar to themselves, and yet corresponding to those which are to be seen in all organized nature. So, also, when the organism is cured the medicine will be no longer absorbed, and that without any injurious consequences so far as general health is concerned.

To resume the conclusions which I have reached, I claim to have established the following facts:

Electro-homœopathy is perfected homœopathy, by the discovery of new therapeutic agents (which I call *electroids*) acting on the blood and giving to the organism the power necessary to cast off the morbid elements which injure it.

This materia medica, like homœopathy of which it is the consummation, has been evolved by experiment, and it rests entirely on facts ascertained by experiment. It it therefore true, and it is simple as truth itself.

Its effects are explained on equally simple principles.

The human body contains principles which are sometimes called herpetic, sometimes scrofulous, or *psoric*, to use Hahnemann's term. Accordingly there are remedies which are *Antiscrofulous.*

These morbid principles often inflict profound injury in the lymph and white corpuscles of the blood. To these we oppose remedies which are *Anticancerous.*

Sometimes this destructive change affects the blood-vessels, the arteries and veins, and the general circulatory system. To this we oppose *Antiangioitic* remedies.

The majority of diseases arise from these three causes, and with these three kinds of remedies we can confront and master them; since, besides their general action on the organism, they have a special and very extended action on different organs, as we shall more fully show subsequently. There are besides, the remedies which belong to their systems. They are—

The *Pectoral* remedies, which act on the bronchial tubes, in the pulmonary system, and catarrhal affections.

The *Febrifuges*, which cure fevers and all types of intermittent diseases, as well as disorders of the liver and the spleen.

The *Antivenereal* remedies cure all forms of syphilis, and even prevent it.

The *Vermifuge* remedies destroy all worms, not only ascarides, but even tœnia and tricocephalis.

Besides these there are liquids having electric properties, which aid the internal cures.

All these remedies are harmless, as may be proved both by analysis and by experience.

Usually the patient takes one globule daily. But if, for the sake of experiment, we administer to any animal whatsoever a hundred, a thousand, any number of globules, no evil results will be observed. Similarly a man may take, without injury, any amount of globules, provided he does not take those which are indicated by some disorder from which he is suffering. Any one who treats himself with these remedies should observe that he can administer several remedies at the same time, not mixing them, but alternating one with another; one remedy for the first half of the day, another for the second.

If there is hæmoptysis—expectoration of blood—a third remedy must be added; that is to say, one of the Angioitics; allotting to each remedy one third part of the day. The rule for the administration of these medicines is, we see, as simple as truth itself. The physician ascertains the cause of a disease, whatever form it may assume; and this is almost always either scrofulous, cancerous, or angioitic. If he has fastened upon the cause, he meets it with the appropriate remedy. For a paralytic case, for instance, the Angioitics are indicated if it proceeds from some obstruction in the circulation; while, if it is caused by psora or scrofula, the anti-scrofolosi must be used.

We facilitate the internal cure by liquids which have electric properties, and which are themselves also designed to combat the cause of the disease. We use the electricity of Angioitic type if the cause exists in the circulatory system. Red Electricity or positive, or else Yellow or negative, or else White or neutral, if the cause is scrofulous. Certain of these electricities, besides their general action, possess also a special specific action, as we shall see when we come to them, and describe the method of using them.

It is well to observe also that the effect which is produced by the internal exhibition of remedies, exists also when they are used externally. A case of hepatitis, for example—inflammation of the liver—will be more quickly subdued if the internal treatment is supplemented by the external use of compresses, or unctions, in the region of the liver and spleen. These external applications are made by using globules of the same remedy which is being used internally; and in doses which will be subsequently indicated.

If a blood-vessel is disordered or altered—as in the case of an aneurism, for example—it will be more quickly cured if the internal treatment is assisted by compresses or unctions applied to the part affected. When grave scrofulous and syphilitic disorders resist treatment by their special remedies, we must have recourse to the *Anticanceroso* remedies.

In fine, when the effect of treatment does not appear, this must proceed from one of the three following causes: Either the initiatory diagnosis is wrong and mistaken remedies are selected, or the dose is wrong; or else the disorganization is so profound that it is impossible by any human means to overcome it. The effect of these remedies is always certain, when they are accurately selected, and rightly applied.

NAMES OF THE REMEDIES AND THEIR GENERAL APPLICATION.

The number of these remedies is thirty-one, of which twenty-six are in globules and five liquid. The latter are called liquid electricities, or simply electricities.

NAMES OF THE GLOBULES, WITH THEIR ABBREVIATIONS.

S.	ANTISCROFOLOSO, or Scrofoloso.	With general constitutional action.
A.	ANTIANGIOITICO, or Angioitico.	
C.	ANTICANCEROSO, or Canceroso.	
F.	FEBRIFUGO.	Special action, but very comprehensive.
Ver.	VERMIFUGO.	
P.	PECTORAL, or Pettorale.	
Ven.	ANTIVENERIEN, or Venereo.	
L.	ANTILYMPHATIC, or Linfatico, often called " the new remedy."	Very general action.

VARIETIES OR HOMONYMES.

S_2	Scrofoloso$_2$, or S. novo.	Wide range of action, but less profound.
S_3	Scrofoloso$_3$ or S. double.	
S_5	Scrofoloso$_5$.	Action extensive and deep.
S_6	Scrofoloso$_6$.	Action less extensive, but deeper.

Scrofoloso Giappone. A febrifuge, and specific for Cholera.

Marina. For eye diseases.

C_2	Canceroso$_2$, or C. novo.	Action extensive and deep.
C_3	Canceroso$_3$, or C. double.	Action less extensive but deeper.
C_4	Canceroso$_4$.	Special action for certain cases.
C	Canceroso .	„ „

C_6	Canceroso$_6$.	Action less extended, but more profound.
C_{10}	Canceroso$_{10}$.	Action less extended, but more profound.
Lord.	Specific in umbilical ruptures.	Action less extended, but more profound.
Dom-fin.	For diphtheria.	Action less extended, but more profound.
T.B.	Canceroso, T.B.	Action less extended, but more profound.
A_2	Angioitico$_2$, or novo.	
A_3	Angioitico$_3$.	Heroic, for certain ca3es.
F_2	Febrifugo$_2$, or novo.	For external use, by compresses to the Hypochondria.
Ver_2	Vermifugo$_2$, or novo.	Action milder and deeper.
P_2	Pettorale$_2$.	Special action.
P_3	Pettorale$_3$.	"
P_4	Pettorale$_4$.	"

The liquids having quasi-electric properties, or more simply *electricities*, are—

Red Electricity.	Positive.
Yellow "	Negative
White "	Neutral, always efficacious.
Blue "	Allied to the Angioitic medicines.
Green "	Negative.

Some recent discoveries on the properties of these electric fluids will be given in a subsequent chapter, treating especially on them.

All the remedies in globule form are taken internally; but it is to be carefully noted that they have an external range of action; and that consequently cure is accelerated by the combined use, external and internal.

Febrifugo$_2$, although generally required for external use, has been very successful as an internal remedy in typhus and grave fevers—in this case it is given in the second dilution. It is necessary always to begin treatment with the first remedies in each series, reserving the varieties for subsequent use when it is proved by experience that the first are insufficient. Thus we see that, with few exceptions, all treatment ought to begin with one of the seven following remedies, viz.:

Scrofoloso, Canceroso, Angioitico, Venereo, Febrifugo, Vermifugo, Pettorale.

It is always understood that when a remedy is named simply, without a qualifying number or name, the first of the series is intended. Thus Scrofoloso is the same as Scrofoloso_1, and so on. This remark is also applicable to the nomenclature employed in the guide books, Vade Mecums—as well as to the labels placed on the bottles.

Among these internal remedies there are three, namely

Scrofoloso, Canceroso, and *Angioitico*,

which take rank as principal or primary remedies. They are pre-eminently the radical medicines in the great majority of cases, the origin of which, as we have repeatedly observed, may be termed Scrofulous, Cancerous, or Angioitic. *Scrofoloso* is applied to disorders or degeneration of the lymph. *Canceroso* to these degenerations when they are grave and advanced, as in cases of cancer and tuberculosis. *Angioitico* is applied to all disorders of the vascular or circulating system.

Among the rest, the varieties, or homonyms, are indicated in special cases. Some of them, as we shall subsequently indicate, have an elective action, for particular types of disease.

These remedies act rapidly, even instantaneously, a circumstance which facilitates experiment in fixing on a remedy. It is, however, to be remarked, that according to peculiarities or idiosyncrasies in different organisms or complications of disease, sensible or distinctly marked effects may be more or less delayed.

Moreover, the blood and the lymph, although belonging to a different system of circulation, and a different set of vessels, have their common origin in the laboratory of digestion, where, in the "storehouse and shop of the whole body," all the materials necessary for the maintenance of life and health are prepared and receive their first start in organization. Consequently, diseases of the lymph may be mixed with disorders of the blood, hence the necessity of frequently resorting to two or more remedies in alternation or succession, in order to make the cure complete.

THE ELECTRICITIES.

I have already sufficiently explained the sense in which the expressions *electric remedies*, *electricities*, are used. Of course we know an electric current has an instantaneous action; that the action of the positive pole is not the same as that of the negative; that the voltaic needle, applied to any point in the course of a nerve, excites it immediately along its entire length, and, by reflex or derived action, the excitement is continued throughout the whole organism. Scientific men, also, who know all this, have invented words to express the effects. They say that the nervous system is in an *electro-tonic* state, a state which the voltaic current has the property of modifying, so as to render it *cat-electrotonic*, or *anelectrotonic*, according to the pole in question. I also have sought words to designate phenomena, hitherto unknown, or which were somewhat mysterious even for myself when I discovered them. When I saw that my liquid remedies acted with a rapidity comparable to that of electricity; when I found that in certain cases they produced a shock; when I saw that on touching the great sympathetic nerve, in its course alongside the seventh cervical vertebra, the whole of the pneumo-gastric tract was influenced; when I obtained the same effect by putting one or more dry globules of *Scrofoloso* on the tongue; finally, when I noticed that one of these liquids would increase tetanic contractions, whilst another would stop them immediately;—when I observed all these facts, and many more of the same class, I said to myself, "Here is electricity—positive, negative, or neutral."

I still cling to these words, and have not yet renounced the idea that there must be in the remedies something which can be called *electroïd* or simply *electric;* or rather we may say that power of this kind is developed from these liquids, and from their contact with the skin where the nerves are nearest the surface,—an electro-motor force, comparable to that which issues from the current of a galvanic pile.

And surely living bodies have their electric-currents! And has not Galvani testified to the existence of a type of animal electricity, which has supplied the celebrated Matteucci with an apparatus comparable to that of an ordinary electric pile? Moreover, is electricity so thoroughly understood that we must believe that it is only to be found in batteries and Leyden jars? Finally, since my electricities are actually contained in the substances from which they are derived, since their action is determined by contact with the skin, I prefer to call these extraordinary remedies, these powerful principles, "*electricities.*"

Formerly, I coloured the electric liquids red, straw-colour, green, blue, &c. I found that this device lent itself to fraudulent imitations; accordingly I no longer colour them. I send out all the electricities colourless, or nearly so, only marking on the labels, *red*, *yellow*, *green*, *blue*, *white;* names which I likewise retain in the nomenclature of the new materia medica.

Electricities are, as a rule, only applied externally, as we shall show; they are often sufficient of themselves for treatment when the disease is only transient, and when there is no internal lesion or organic change. This is the case in a multitude of simple maladies. It would be wrong to conclude from this that they are simply palliatives. Generally, the electricities, if skilfully administered, supply a powerful auxiliary in the entire treatment of a disorder, which, for its absolute cure, requires also internal remedies.

GENERAL INDICATIONS FOR THE USE OF THE ELECTRO-HOMŒOPATHIC REMEDIES.

The electro-homœopathic remedies produce a gentle action, often instantaneous but generally progressive, and such that the obvious effects are evident only after a certain period has elapsed; this period is only a few minutes in acute cases, and several days in deep-seated chronic disorders. In this, again, there is an analogy between the remedy and the course of the disease.

The instantaneous action of the remedies can be ascertained by giving several globules of Scrofoloso dry to any person seized with a fainting fit, threatened with paralysis, troubled with seasickness, dysentery, &c.: the disorder will be instantly dissipated. By means of a few globules of Scrofoloso, I have sometimes rendered intoxicated persons immediately sober.

I have also seen hysterical, convulsive, and angioitic persons faint at the contact of red or yellow electricity; when eight or ten globules of Scrofoloso dry, have uniformly remedied this at once.

It is the same thing at the threatening of cholera, diphtheria, stomach disorder, indigestion, &c. The purification of the blood, in the majority of cases, is seen by the elimination of the morbid and foreign bodies which are driven from the organism, in some cases by free perspiration, by expectoration, or by deposits in the urine; in others, by the appearance of a crop of boils, or by a crisis of diarrhœa, which is neither alarming nor painful.

It is especially in cases of wounds, aneurisms, tumours, and pains, that external remedies must be used. It must be remembered, however, that the external use of our remedies is but auxiliary to the internal treatment, and that, as the treatment advances, the dose must be increased to render the effect more powerful. The reverse is the case with the internal remedies.

SPHERE OF ACTION OF THE REMEDIES.

THE SCROFOLOSO GROUP.

The Scrofoloso series, particularly 1 and 5, are the most remarkable for their power, and for the extent of their sphere of action. Their action is to antidote the psoric, herpetic, and scrofulous principles, with which we are told the organism is more or less impregnated. These principles, by their nature, accumulate in quantity, and augment in force continually, and must in time produce serious weakness or premature old age. The action of the remedies, when sufficiently prolonged, drives them out of the body. This is the reason that nine diseases out of ten are cured by these medicines, which is proved by experience; whence it may be concluded that the majority of diseases arise from the *scrofula* which, according to our theory, is one of the products of hereditary lepra or syphilis.

It is for this reason that the Scrofoloso medicines prevent disease. The other remedies nip disease in the bud, but do not completely anticipate it; whilst the Scrofoloso group, in purifying the psoric constitution, prevent disease from appearing; they not only kill germs, but they make the soil in which they germinate no longer capable of developing them.

Only the Scrofoloso remedies, therefore, can be taken for preventive purposes, to make the body secure from the assault of disease, to establish health by means of sound digestion, quiet and refreshing sleep; providing against tendency to chills, fluxions, innumerable slight disorders, which are, for the most part, the starting-points of graver diseases.

Whole families and even populations can place themselves as it were out of reach of many diseases, and can constantly renew their security by the habitual use of Scrofoloso, mixed with their food or the water which they drink.

Scrofoloso has also a special action on the following disorders: Myelitis, or inflammation of the spine, acute or chronic, with consequent paralysis of the sphincters of the anus or bladder; sciatica; chronic conjunctivitis, catarrhal ophthalmia, or else rheumatic, scrofulous, epidemic or endemic ophthalmia; lachrymal fistula; granular, contagious, or purulent conjunctivitis; commencing cataract; thickening of the optic membranes, with feebleness or loss of sight; otalgia, chronic mucous disorder of the exterior meatus; purulent otorrhœa, deafness; acoustic hallucinations; coryza; ozœna; scrofulous inflammation of the nasal passages; perverted sense of smell; acute and chronic stomatitis; fistula of the salivary ducts; increase of salivary secretion; fistula of the gums; suppression or exaggeration of taste; acute or chronic angina (alternating with the Angioitics); erysipelas, phlegmonous, epidemic, exanthemic; hypertrophy of the tonsils; hydrophobia; croup; ordinary and herpetic laryngitis; hoarseness; gastric irritation, gastralgia, hiccup, dyspepsia, chronic or mucous gastritis, produced by the retrocession of a herpetic eruption; indigestion, flatulency, acidity of the stomach, nervous and spasmodic; sea-sickness;

pancreatitis; constipation; diarrhœa, serous and epidemic; painter's or lead colic; tenesmus of the rectum; putrid intestinal fevers (alternating with Febrifugo); gastro-enteric fever with miliary eruption (alternating with Febrifugo), or with extension of disease to brain; hernia; spasmodic contraction of the hernial sac; humoral diathesis consequent on grave disorder attacking the digestive apparatus; blenorrhœa of the rectum; acute and chronic nephritis, or inflammation of the kidneys; nephralgia, original or symptomatic; diabetes; albuminuria; suppuration and abscess in the kidneys; affections of the ureters; acute and chronic cystitis (alternating with the Angioitics); catarrh of the bladder; gravel (Scrofoloso is heroic in these cases); hydrocele; spermatorrhœa; involuntary pollutions; prostatitis; urethral neuralgia; itch, herpes of all kinds, impetigo, profuse foot-sweat, rheumatism, gout, acute and chronic disorders of the lymphatics; adenitis; inflammation of lymphatic glands in the neck, the throat, and the groin; goitre, &c.

THE ANGIOITIC GROUP.

These remedies are the regulators and purifiers of the blood; they act on the whole of the circulatory system, and especially on the heart and all its disorders. Since impurity of the blood entails corresponding impurity in the lymph, and *vice versa*, it is often necessary to alternate the Angioitics with the Scrofoloso or Canceroso group, or with special remedies. Thus, when in certain changes of the sanguinary system, such as varicosity, hypertrophy of the heart, &c., there occurs at the same time congestion of the liver, for which Febrifugo is specific, Angioitico will be alternated with Febrifugo, either internally or externally.

When the electricities applied externally have no effect, some grave change in the blood or circulation must be suspected. In this case compresses, unctions, and baths of Angioitico will be substituted with advantage.

Besides this general action, these remedies possess a special action on the following pathological conditions:

Cerebral congestion, active or passive; acute or chronic meningitis; encephalitis; vertigo and congestive headache; lethargy; somnolence arising from inflammation or congestion of the brain; trismus and spasms of the muscles of the eyes, the face, the mouth, the tongue, when they are symptomatic of cerebral inflammation; acute attacks of monomania, and in general all sorts of mental disorder; sunstroke; idiopathic or traumatic apoplexy with effusion of blood, and paralysis of one or both sides; acute and chronic pneumonia; pulmonary arteritis; simple pleurisy (with these three disorders the Pectoral remedies must be alternated); congestion of the lungs; pericarditis;

carditis; acute or chronic endocarditis; hydro-pericarditis; steno-carditis; fainting; syncope; cardiac congestion or apoplexy; palpitation; aneurisms, and other organic lesions of the heart; inflammation of the thoracic or abdominal aorta; general arteritis; angina pectoris; acute inflammatory fevers (alternating with Febrifugo), phlebitis, functional or traumatic; varicose disorders, &c.

THE CANCEROSO GROUP.

These remedies manifest their specific action against all scrofulous disorders when they reach their gravest and most advanced stages; such as scirrhus, passive tumours, &c., which, for this reason, resist the action of Scrofoloso.

The cure of scirrhus and cancer is certain so long as the vital organs are not too profoundly affected, or so long as the loss of strength, the encroachment of the disease, and the rapidity of its course, have not arrived at such a point that there is no time left for the remedy to purify the blood. This is especially the case when the fever attending absorption has commenced. In this extreme case, the certainty of cure is lost; but not the certainty of giving relief, of diminishing or removing pain and postponing the fatal result. But it is said—

Principiis obsta, sero medicina paratur
Quum mala per longas invaluere moras;

which means that evil must be combated at its commencement, and that we must not wait until the patient is moribund, or till cure is impossible.

The first effect of the Canceroso is often to seem to distinctly increase the disease; the reason is to be found in the action of the remedy itself, which stirs the depths of the organism in order to expel the cancerous principles and separate in some way the living parts from those which are already in the conditions of dead or foreign bodies.

Sometimes also the good effect seems to be delayed or stationary, during the period necessary for the remedy to penetrate and saturate, so to speak, the organism. But as soon as this saturation point is attained, the cure commences, and proceeds with ever augmenting rapidity. The treatment of these diseases may last for months, sometimes for years; more or less time, according to the disease which has to be conquered. Exceptional difficulties may present themselves, the disease may be at a standstill, or even sustain partial relapse; but there need be no discouragement, perseverance will certainly in time remove it if that is humanly possible; for the remedies do not deceive and their effect is assured.

In cancer, as soon as cure has commenced, treatment must never be interrupted; relapses, often irreparable, may occur. I say this with a full knowledge of the cause, and it is most important to fix this condition well in the mind.

The Cancerosos which are most effectual in the treatment of cancer are—Canceroso$_1$, Canceroso$_4$, Canceroso$_5$.

The Cancerosos are also specific against spasms of the womb, laborious accouchements, cancers, tumours, and indurations of the ovaries; serous or mucous metritis; acute and chronic discharges; leucorrhœa; uterine polypi; hypertrophy of the os, or neck of the uterus; acute and chronic vaginitis; vaginal fistula; suppuration and abscess of the mammary glands; scirrhus and other cancers in the breast; ascites; ovaritis; tumours of various kinds.

Canceroso$_2$ has a gentler and deeper action; it is especially useful in dropsy.

Canceroso$_4$ has a special action against cancer, and especially against diseases of the bones: such as acute and chronic osteitis; osteo-myelitis; inflammation of the joints; coxalgia; inflammatory diseases of the hip, the knee, the ankle, and various regions of the vertebral column; caries and necrosis of the bones; osteal neuralgia or disorders when they do not arise from syphilis; periostitis; panaris, whitlow, &c.

Canceroso$_5$ has a much more profound and special action on the pulmonary organs than the other Cancerosos, and it is the one mostly used externally.

Cancerso$_{10}$ is a combination of the cancerous remedies.

The Febrifugos 1 and 2.

List of the principal disorders against which these specifics may be employed.

Intermittent and periodic diseases; quotidian, tertian, and quartan agues; simple and complicated periodic fevers; pernicious fevers; intermittent neuralgias, such as intermittent *tic douloureux*, intermittent headache; nervous disorders which spread from the nervous centres to the abdominal and thoracic ganglions of the sympathetic nerve; cardiac neuroses, with palpitations; suffocation or nervous dyspnœa; various magnetic conditions, as ecstasy, somnambulism, spontaneous clairvoyance, consequent upon some nervous disturbance in the solar plexus or semilunar ganglions; hysterical or ovarian nervous attacks; morbid conditions in various functions of organic or vegetative life; affections of the liver or spleen, such as acute or chronic hepatitis, chronic enlargement or congestion of the liver, jaundice, acute and chronic splenitis, hypochondria, &c.

Nature, which ever aims at the grandest results, has placed the centre of will and intellect, the forces that govern movement and sensation, in the brain and spinal cord; but it has also provided a system of nervous supply whose office it is to watch over that class of phenomena which are continuously proceeding in the organism; that is to say, the functions of organic nutrition and decomposition, of repair and separation. This system of nerve supply can act independently and even without the cognizance of the central, cerebro-spinal system to which is allotted the higher functions of life. What a source of weariness and disgust for the nobler faculties—for intellect, thought, emotion, will—if these higher order of functions had to watch perpetually over the lower necessities of vegetative and organic life. The independent vitality of the involuntary part of nervous energy has been well illustrated by the memorable labours of the illustrious Bichat.

Accordingly the wisdom of Nature has provided a special nervous system, called the sympathetic, or the visceral, or splanchnic nerves, placed alongside the vertebral column, starting by anastomosis with the optic ganglion, and continued from the summit to the base of the spinal column. This is a collection of nerve filaments, interspersed with ganglions, and forming constantly plexuses of nerves, inosculating with the nerves of the spinal and cerebral system, which govern motion, sensation, and reflex action. These nerves also encircle the large thoracic and abdominal arteries, forming a kind of sheath; they also follow them in their course throughout the body, conveying nervous power, the breath of life on which nutrition depends.

The eye is strongly influenced by the optic

ganglion; the organ of hearing, all the organs in the neck, such as the throat and the larynx, are governed by plexuses of nerves and filaments from the cervical ganglions. The heart, the aorta, and the lungs also by a network of filaments, which form so many considerable plexuses. How many morbid nervous conditions are occasioned by disorder in the semilunar glands and the solar plexus, whose power, or susceptibility, in nervous persons, attains such a height that they are almost equivalent to a secondary cerebral system, which is perhaps the seat of some forms of intuition, and gives rise to the phenomena of clairvoyance. How many neuralgias, neuroses, and psychical disorders are developed, especially in nervous women, of a delicate or finely strung temperament, by disorders of the solar plexus. Doubtless these considerations influenced Stahl in assigning to this plexus the seat of the soul itself, and Van-Helmont in pointing to this as the central principle of life. On both sides of the abdominal spine down to the extreme end—the coccyx—we may see distributed innumerable filaments and ganglions of the sympathetic nerve. On one side these filaments branch off to the digestive organs and the urino-genital system; on the other, they join and inosculate with the other filaments from the spinal system, and thus are distributed over the abdominal blood-vessels, and follow them to their destination in the limbs.

When the sensations which depend upon this secondary nervous system are not too violent, they do not pass out of their proper *loci;* but if they are too acutely strung, they pass outside their physiological enclosure and act upon the cerebro-spinal system, and create in the mind a conscious perception of the disorder that has visited the vegetative sphere; rather they constitute what we may term a splanchnopathic disease, or a morbid condition of the sympathetic or ganglionic system.

The morbid phenomena of the great visceral, or splanchnic nerve, and the sympathetic reflex symptoms which are produced outside its sphere in the different organs of the body, require much diagnostic tact in the physician in order that they may be recognized and understood: but the clinically educated eye soon learns to distinguish them, and to discriminate in general symptoms those which depend on local disorder, and those which arise by reflex action from disease of the sympathetic system. Certain kinds of diplopia, or double vision—especially in helminthiasis, or worm diseases, with dilatation of the pupil and blue circles round the eyes—certain cases of amaurosis, or blindness, accompanied with impaired nutrition and weakness in digestive functions, proceed, very often, from some deep affection of the sympathetic nerves. Certain nervous spasms of the throat and larnyx, oppression in breathing without inflammatory or organic cause—attacks of fainting or syncope, palpitations of the heart when not dependent upon organic or antecedent disease of that organ—have also their source in a neuropathic change in the functional filaments or ganglions, or in some of the plexuses of the visceral nerves.

In undertaking the treatment of these vague and indefinite conditions, we must always begin with some doses of Angioitico or Scrofoloso, according to the constitution of the patient; and if this treatment does not succeed, we shall no doubt be more fortunate if we resort to Febrifugo$_1$ internally, and compresses of Febrifugo$_2$ to the hypochondria.

All those disorders of the solar plexus which we have referred to, as spontaneous somnambulism, ecstasy, various grades of morbid sensibility (that sensibility or sentimentalism which exists in infinite variety in those unhappy women whose state baffles all pathological classification—*femmes incomprises*); also some psychical disorders of the solar plexus, as hypochondriasis; also nostalgia, pining or home sickness, require the use of the specific which is now under consideration. Very often catalepsy is provoked by a morbid exaltation of sensibility in the solar plexus. Therefore we must combat it with this specific, continuing the treatment for a long time in order to prevent the return of a disease which may easily degenerate into epilepsy. But I will not dwell on these recognized disorders, whose multitudinous and protean varieties and gradations demand a consideration which is perhaps more philosophic than practical. I prefer to speak of an order of affections with which we are only too familiar, which constantly come under medical observation, which are endemic in certain localities, although they may appear in all kinds of climate and position without exception —I mean intermittent fevers, simple, complicated, or pernicious.

It is an axiom of pathological science, and the anatomical and physiological reasons for it are incontrovertible, that periodic disorders generally, and intermittent fevers in particular depend upon a neuropathic state of the great sympathetic or ganglionic nerve, accompanied with a more or less marked change in the circulation and the gastro-enteric system. Whatever may be the machinery which nature employs to give rise to an attack of fever, we shall never be at a loss for fixing upon its primary cause as soon as we recognize the teaching of anatomy and physiology, that the sympathetic or visceral nerve is distributed over the great central artery, the aorta, and from thence to every artery and capillary of the body: that the circulation of the blood is everywhere controlled by the sympathetic nerve. This it is that explains the shivering, the retarded circulation, the arrested pulse, the goose-flesh, which arise at the beginning of the attack, or the spasmodic stage in the sympathetic nerves—the heat or perspiration with augmented circulation in the period of reaction, since reaction always follows primary action. But the most important point is, that a vigorous treatment which cures these affections does not leave the sad consequences which are always to be found in the progress of intermittent fevers, as ordinarily treated.

The profound and yet gentle action of the Febrifugo medicines attacks the morbid cause directly, but does not produce any of the terrible effects which result from the indiscriminating use of the crowd of remedies which are employed against these fevers.

As soon as an attack of fever has been broken, it will not be prudent to be satisfied with this measure of success; but the use of Febrifugo must be still continued for some time, in order to eradicate the morbid cause existing in an abnormal action of the fibres of the sympathetic nerve, and in order to prevent the relapses which so often occur in these diseases. It will be also advisable, whenever this can be managed, to remove the patient for some time from the locality where the intermittent fever has been contracted.

The clinically practised eye will easily distinguish between the simple suspension of periodic attacks and radical cure. In the first case, although the attack no longer returns, yet he does not experience the same buoyant and elastic health which he formerly enjoyed. The pulse is wiry and feeble; the tongue has a dirty, yellowish coating, showing that the morbid germ is still lurking in the organism, and that the use of the Febrifugo must be continued, in alternation sometimes with Scrofoloso, or Angioitico, according to the constitution of the patient. It often happens that intermittent fevers are followed by some secondary and chronic disorder—such as congestion of the liver, the spleen, or the mesentery; infirmities of digestion, general inflation or local swelling in the abdomen. The specifics Scrofoloso and Canceroso, continued for a long time, will ultimately disperse all these troublesome survivals or relics of a half-cured disease. These sequent miseries are reserved for those unfortunate persons who are treated by large doses of quinine, administered by doctors who think they can cure an attack of ague, or intermittent fever, by suppressing its periodic returns by this remedy, which, being so valuable, ought always to be used with careful selection, since it is always injurious when a preliminary course of treatment is not resorted to in order to subdue the central disorder, which is of the nature of a distinct gastro-enteric disturbance.

Slow fevers, gastro-enteritis, with swelling or feeling of distension in the stomach after food, with breaking up of the constituents of the blood, the cause of abdominal dropsy or dropsy of the limbs, or general dropsical swelling (anasarca), are almost always the consequences of this mischievous practice of suppressing periodic attacks of fever, without heed to their complications.

Electro-Homœopathy, which is at once powerful in its action and rational in its operation, removes all these complications, and then cures the morbid cause by acting on the source of the evil; and consequently the growing grounds of the periodic attacks. Sometimes cinchona, employed in the usual and well-known manner, is only capable of suspending the periodic returns of fever for a few days; or if it succeeds, it is only for a short time and at the cost of grave danger to the organism. It is especially in these refractory cases, which are extremely prevalent in certain localities, that my remedies achieve such splendid results. But if it is desired to banish the disease entirely, it is imperative on the physician and the patient to persevere persistently in the use of the Febrifugos, in order that a sort of periodic habit which the ganglionic system contracts, may be shaken off.

Intermittent fevers in general, and pernicious fevers in particular, result from the poisonous action of a miasma which is diffused in the air, known under the name of marsh miasm. It is generated in marshy districts by the decomposition of vegetable and animal substances. In this point of view the miasm of cholera may be brought into comparison with the marsh miasma, with this difference however, that the latter attacks more particularly the ganglionic nervous system, while the former aims its deadly blows at the entire nervous system —the cerebro-spinal system and that great and essential division of the cerebral system called the pneumo-gastric nerve, which, in my view, is the point of contact between organic life and the higher and reflex system.

I have seen congestions, enlargements, obstructions, and enormous and obstinate indurations of the hepatic substance, disappear under the action of the Febrifugos. When given at the commencement, before the disease has completely established itself, they are capable of stamping it out; and when they cannot entirely expel it they certainly relieve and moderate its violence.

Compresses and unctions of Febrifugo$_2$ over the splenic region give excellent results in all kinds of weakness or disease. This by itself indicates the importance of this viscus, the exact use of which has not yet been discovered by physiologists. Indeed there is more than one dark corner in science which will be illuminated by the light reflected on them by the new remedies. The classic divisions of diseases, for instance, have no real value in many cases, if we judge of their nature by the effects of the Scrofolosos, which clearly demonstrate the fact that a crowd of diseases which apparently have nothing in common, may be traceable to one origin.

Vermifugos 1 and 2.

These are employed against all worm affections without exception—from ascarides to tœnia and tricocephalus. Forty or fifty globules in a glass of water may sometimes be properly taken. When a disease, especially a chronic disease, resists the specific which is proper to it, it is well to give a dose of vermifugo; since the presence of intestinal worms may frequently destroy or prevent the action of the remedies.

Pectoral 1.

This is specific for the following disorders: Irritation of the mucous membrane of the bronchi and trachea; acute and chronic bronchitis; capillary and follicular bronchitis; tracheitis and bronchitis caused by sulphurous vapours; bronchorrhœa, and in general all disorders of the bronchial tubes.

Pectoral 2.

This is a powerful specific for the following disorders: Pulmonary inflammation; pneumorrhagia, or pulmonary flux symptomatic of tubercular softening; tubercular phthisis; slow or galloping consumption; pulmonary emphysema, or dilatation of the air-cells.

Pectoral 3 and 4.

These are indicated in catarrhal flux of the bronchial mucous membrane, chronic catarrh, and the suffocating catarrh of old people; and in all kinds of cough.

THE NEW REMEDY, OR LINFATICO

(RECENTLY INTRODUCED).

This has a universal action both on the blood and on the lymph. It is used, in preference, externally; by baths, unctions, and compresses.

VENEREO.

Syphilitic Infection.—May occur directly, or by any method by which any exposed or mucous surface may come in contact with another. The virus may be conveyed by other objects—a cigar, a spoon, a bath, &c.

The time necessary between contagion and the development of symptoms may be 24 or 48 hours; or from one to three weeks. As a rule, symptoms appear between the third and sixth day after exposure to infection.

Early Symptoms.—After any impure contact, the human system may be infected by different poisons, which differ distinctly in their symptoms, progress, and consequences. One of them is the syphilitic poison; the other is gonorrhœa, or blenorrhœa, which may appear in various mucous surfaces (as the eye), besides locally.

Syphilitic Infection.—Manifests itself as virulent ulcer, or primary bubo, in the first instance. This may lead to phymosis or paraphymosis, *i.e.*, swelling which makes either re-traction or pro-traction of the prepuce impossible. Another primary form is that of blenorrhœa, or urethral flux.

Secondary or Constitutional Symptoms.—In this case bubo, or inflammation of the glands of the groin, follows the closure of the primary ulcers, especially if they have been suppressed by cauterization. Orchitis may arise from the same cause; enlargement of the cervical glands; ulcerative disease in the throat and its vicinity; baldness; ophthalmia of the two varieties; skin disorders, pustular, papular, encrusted; mucous tubercles, &c.

Tertiary Symptoms, or Syphilitic Cachexia.—Among these we must include disorders of the bones in their substance or coverings; fibrous neuralgias; and as the last result of fully developed constitutional invasion, venereal consumption.

Blenorrhagic Infection.—The results of gonorrhœal infection are urethral inflammation of various kinds—torpid, erysipelatous, chordee, or violent tension; phymosis in its two forms; balanitis, excrescences or growths which Hahnemann called sycosis, and which are familiarly termed crests or cauliflower growths. Subsequently, if discharge has been suppressed by astringents, organic changes in the canal.

Venereo, or the anti-syphilitic specific, must

always be the basis of the treatment, but it must be alternated with Angioitico when phagedenic or gangrenous complications arise, caused by exuberant vascularity; or with Scrofoloso when the cause of complication may be traced to mucous irritation of the digestive system, or gastric disorder. Also Canceroso must be used in serpiginous or herpetic varieties.

Treatment of Primary Ulceration.—In treating the original ulcer we must look to the three primary conditions which meet and embody themselves in the disease so as to constitute its real essence. 1. That condition which is common to a great number of diseases, *i.e.*, ulcerative inflammation, producing a solution of continuity in the skin and mucous membranes. 2. The objective condition, in the presence of virulent pus secreted by an artificial membrane of a specific character, a structure *sui generis*—a newly formed pyogenic apparatus. 3. The dynamic results of this virus in the organism, that is its capability of lodgment in every part of the body from crown to sole. We are thus confronted by three capital conditions, which cannot be ignored by any one who desires to effect a radical cure of the primary ulcer, and to feel secure that his patient is rescued by therapeutic treatment from general infection. In the treatment of the primary ulcer we must for some days use Angioitico; it will dissipate the general symptoms which arise from local poisoning and the consequent revolt of the vital forces to the invading force—such symptoms as heaviness of the head, insomnia, heat of the skin, loss of appetite, and that indefinable *malaise* which is felt by every one thus attacked. At the same time this remedy will check ulcerative inflammation, and arrest the vascular congestion which is formed around the central venereal injury.

In this way the liability to internal and external inflammation is removed, and the danger is averted of phagedenic or gangrenous ulceration. Angioitico must be continued for three or four days to check and reduce inflammation in the ulcer, and to limit its extension. Thus the first condition of treatment is met.

The second process, which must proceed *pari passu* with the first, consists in eliminating the syphilitic virus. We take 25 globules of Venereo, and dissolve it in six ounces of water ; a piece of lint must be soaked in this solution and applied to the ulcer, as soon as it appears, or as soon as treatment begins. This application, which should be repeated four times a day, should be continued till red granulations appear at the base of the ulcer, that is till it is thoroughly clean and assumes a state favourable to cicatrization. By this method the syphilitic virus is completely destroyed, by applying the antidote to the place where it is first deposited, and thus it is prevented from penetrating into the deeper recesses of the body. Our belief is that this material application acts only on the grosser parts of the virus, and that its finer constituents are able to evade its operation. In order to fit the nature and modifications of the virus we believe that a third process is necessary ; after five or six external applications of the Venereo the same remedy must be taken internally, both in dilution and in dry globules, as follows : The first day, two globules after food morning and evening ; the second day, three globules morning and evening ; the next day five ; and so on until we reach ten globules after food, or twenty daily. Then the same graduated series is reversed—that is, we diminish the dose daily till we return to the original dose. Immersion baths, in which 100 or 150 globules of the same specific are dissolved, will much facilitate cure. If this treatment is rigorously followed, we may be assured that all the necessities of the case, as a contagious disease, are met.

Serpiginous or Herpetic Ulceration.—It may be that, in spite of following these directions exactly, the ulcer may resist cicatrization. This usually arises from a herpetic taint which disturbs the normal course of the disease. This state of things will be met, after using Angioitico and Venereo, by the use of Scrofoloso 1 and 5, which, by removing the herpetic complications, will hasten cicatrization.

Phagedenic or Gangrenous Ulcer and Bubo.—Sometimes, either on account of the general condition of the vital secretions throughout the body, or from some local vascular inflammation in the intestines, generally gastro-enteric, which is reflected in the morbid condition of the skin locally, the bubo or ulceration may be attacked by violent inflammation, of so malignant a quality as to assume a gangrenous type and constitute a phagedenic ulcer.

The best way of preventing this serious complication is to continue the use of Angioitico, alternately with the Cancerosos, 1 and 5, in dilution, and to take dry globules of the same. We advise also the use of compresses on the ulcer or bubo, of $Canceroso_5$ and Green Electricity, which will allay pain; at the same time the corresponding nerves should be treated with alternate applications of Red and Yellow Electricity.

There is another disorder which may result from the primary symptoms of syphilis, or from blenorrhagia; and that is orchitis, or inflammation of the testicle. This disease, which may fix the patient to a bed of suffering for months together, is relieved in a surprising degree, and in a very short time, by Electro-Homœopathy. Although cure must be effected by Venereo, we must employ $Angioitico_3$ much attenuated, alternated with the Scrofolosos, and the results will be truly surprising. Attention to diet, rest, refreshing beverages, must also be combined with the use of specifics.

Treatment of Constitutional Syphilis.—When we have to combat the secondary symptoms of syphilitic infection—such as swelling of various glands, ulcers in the throat or larynx, with hoarseness or loss of voice, mucous or purulent expectoration—we must never forget that although the disease is derived from a specific principle, and is sustained by it, it is attended by an inflammatory element, and by disorders which affect all the vital functions. Here it is that Angioitico and the Scrofolosos evidently find their application. Indeed, after the centres of chronic inflammation are quieted, and gastric or herpetic complications removed—since these specifics, answering to the governing generic characteristics of human diseases, are composed of a number of simple agents capable of meeting all gradations of disease by dynamic and effective antidotes—nothing can be more natural than that Venereo should show its efficacy on the organism which has been to a great extent purified of counteracting influences. If, however, we wish to be assured that the patient is entirely cured of general syphilitic contagion, the use of Venereo must be continued for three or four months. If this treatment has been continued during the autumn or to the beginning of winter, it may be resumed at spring-time for forty days, for at that period the actively vital fluids and forces stir into activity also those portions of the virus which are most deeply rooted in the organism. Although ordinary anti-syphilitic treatment, such as mercurial ointment and friction, and the internal use of various mercurial preparations, may cause the syphilitic symptoms to disappear for some time and even sometimes cure them, it is no less certain that the use of these therapeutic agents may lead to very disastrous results. They enfeeble the most vigorous constitutions, and the most robust bodies are reduced to shadow. But—and this is still worse—after having corrupted the organism, mercury produces its own diseases, salivation, stomatitis, glossitis, eczema, &c., during which time venereal symptoms disappear, but are not cured. And it may be after a considerable lapse of time, when mercurial effects have ceased, these same symptoms may assume other forms, out of their protean list, and, unfortunately, may take the form of monomania.

I.—*Syphilitic Conjunctivitis.*—The distinctive characteristic of this disease is a vascular zone, which surrounds the cornea with a ring of a reddish coppery tint. It gives rise to sympathetic symptoms in the lachrymal gland, and in the trigeminal (or facial) nerves, producing lachrymation, and considerable supra- and sub-orbital neuralgia.

II. — *Syphilitic Iritis.* — This disease is characterized by a strong contraction of the pupil, with immobility of the iris, which swells outwardly, and approaches the posterior surface of the cornea. This membrane loses its normal colour and is injected with blood, like the eyes of a tiger. The condylomata formed may destroy the structure of the iris, or cause adhesion between it and the cornea. Lachrymation is attended with neuralgic pains in and around the orbit. When this kind of ophthalmia arises, it must be treated promptly: for one day's delay may deprive the patient of one of the most precious endowments of life.

During two days, the specific, Scrofoloso or Angioitico, adapted to the constitution of the patient must be given. With this remedy, local bathing with the Angioitics or Scrofolosos; frequent application of Blue or Red Electricity, alternated with Yellow upon, above, and below the orbits, to the occiput and the great sympathetic nerve. After this, the selected specific must be alternated with Venereo, until the eye ceases to be painfully affected by light, and all the subjective and objective symptoms have completely disappeared.

If we study with some carefulness the pathological history of disease, we may always follow a primary infection step by step till it assumes the form either of rash or of chronic ophthalmia. Hygienic care of the skin should be intelligently attended to. What we especially advise is the use of immersion baths which can at once secure cleanliness and strengthen all local and general curative processes.

Diseases of the osseous and fibrous systems; bone pains; inflammation, caries, and necrosis of the bones.

Tertiary Syphilis.—The distinctive character of

the sufferings attendant upon tertiary syphilis is that they begin during the evening, become ameliorated to a slight extent for two hours before mid-night, and reappear with renewed and wearisome force for the two following hours. This is the course of nocturnal osseous pains. Any bone in the body may be thus seized: the tibia, femur, carpal and tarsal bones, the sternum, and all the bony sympheses and crests, all may suffer. But the venereal virus appears to select the gelatinous substance for its most determined assaults. Thus it settles on the laryngeal cartilages, especially the epiglottis; also on the cartilaginous ends of spongy bones where gelatine is most abundant.

Hydrargyrosis, or Mercurial Disease.—There has never been any discovery, however good, which has not, in this evil world, been warped from its proper use, and made an instrument of death, disease, and degradation to man. This has happened with mercury. Wisely administered, this medicine is not dangerous; on the contrary, it has a specific action in antidoting venereal virus. But if taken in large doses, as we usually find it prescribed in our time, it acts upon the organic tissues and on the secretions of the body in the same way as the syphilitic poison. For it acts upon the lymphatic system, producing glandular swellings; upon the gastro-enteric mucous membranes, producing bad forms of intestinal inflammation, dysentery, &c.; upon the mucous surfaces of the throat and mouth and gums, producing the mercurial stomatitis and glossitis, attended with profuse salivation. These things are so well known that we need not dwell upon them. The abuse of mercury may even cause pulmonary phthisis and apoplexy. The skin also is attacked by a peculiar mercurial disease, called eczema, resembling the idiopathic variety of the same disease. But the most serious effects of mercury are seen in the periostitis produced in the osseous and fibrous structures; ostitis, caries, necrosis, with decay and discoloration of the teeth. The substance of the brain itself is not exempt from liability to mercurial disease; numerous cases are recorded of insanity, facial neuralgia, *delirium tremens* which have arisen in the course of syphilitic disease when it has been maltreated by massive doses of mercurial preparations, and especially of corrosive sublimate. The spinal marrow shares the evil; slow myelitis, with trembling or tremors of the limbs, impossibility of writing or walking steadily, are familiar results. The whole mass of the blood is deeply affected; its plasticity reduced, and its composition altered. Hence arise serous effusion in the pleuritic cavity, the pericardium and the peritoneum, and œdema and anasarca are not infrequent.

Whenever we are called to treat a patient who has been thus mismanaged, the first thing to be done is to abandon entirely the use of the mercurials which have created the condition of hydrargyrosis, or mercurial disease, and administer the electro-homœopathic remedy which his constitution requires. With this, Venereo must be alternated, which will at once meet the bad effects of mercurial treatment, and completely destroy the venereal taint. It is scarcely necessary to add that the *régime* in this artificial disease, which is so analogous to ordinary venereal disease, must be attended to in the same way, by regulating diet and hygienic management.

TREATMENT OF GONORRHŒA AND ITS RESULTS.

The symptoms of acute gonorrhœa are well known; and we need not occupy ourselves by minute description: we shall concern ourselves chiefly with its treatment by the new method.

The prognosis of this disease is much more favourable, in our opinion, when it begins with an acute and painful stage, than when it assumes an indolent and well-nigh non-inflammatory condition; since in the latter case the struggle between the disease and the remedy will be entered upon with difficulty, the salutary reactions will be slow, and there is a danger lest it should be converted into a lingering or interminable chronic flux. The medical man is fortunate who is called to treat such a case during its acute stage, before treatment has begun, or he has made any use of any one of those many agencies which are so prejudicial. In this case he may reckon upon not having to deal with secondary or chronic conditions, resulting from the acute attack.

During the first four or five days of treatment Angioitico is naturally most in requisition. When the smarting and inflammatory symptoms are considerably diminished, and the gonorrhœal flux has commenced, and the attendant nervous condition reduced, Angioitico must be alternated with Venereo, and applications of Blue Electricity, or Red, alternated with Yellow, according to the patient's type, must be made to the pubic region, the perinæum, and the great sympathetic nerve; and once a day the patient must take internally 5 or 10 drops of Yellow Electricity in a teaspoonful of water. Treatment must not be discontinued until the flux has entirely ceased—it need scarcely be noted that all astringent injections are interdicted in our treatment. The functions must be carried on without the least pain, and we must be well assured that the purulent secretion has completely disappeared owing to the interior and specific action of our remedies.

It is better that gonorrhœa should go through its several stages with some deliberation rather than stop suddenly; for this would not be a cure, but simply a suppression of the flow, and a source of great danger to adjacent or related organs. A moderate diet, perfect rest at the beginning of the disease, the use of a suspensory bandage for the testicle, are indispensable in order to secure a favourable result.

Gonorrhœal Rheumatism.—Among the unfortunate consequences of suppressed gonorrhœa we must reckon gonorrhœal rheumatism. This disease begins with pain and swelling in the articulations of the knees and feet, and is manifested also by intense pain in the shoulders without redness or swelling. Sometimes, also, these rheumatic pains have not any fixed character, but wander from one point to another in the fibrous structures of the lower extremities, and often prove a source of torment to age when youth has been wild and stormy. If we are called upon to treat acute rheumatism in its violent stage, which is most usually accompanied by all the symptoms of vascular reaction, we must for some days, as before, make use of Angioitico, and subsequently administer Venereo. But it may be that the disease has taken such a firm hold on the fibrous tissues that it will be necessary to alternate Angioitico and Canceroso. Whenever chronic rheumatic troubles have to be treated, and the latent presence of any venereal disorder is suspected, it is best to begin at once the alternate use of Venereo and Canceroso.

Gonorrhœal Ophthalmia: or Ocular Blenorrhagia.—This is another terrible disease which unfortunately is but too often the consequence of attempting to suppress gonorrhœa without curing it. It is a terrible disease, of a violently inflammatory type, which is capable of destroying the eye in a short time by rapid suppuration. It will be necessary then to arrest the progress of the evil by the most energetic treatment, for the disorganization of the eye is always the unhappy consequence of neglected or ineffectual treatment.

Urinary Obstruction, or Stricture.—This is another evil result of gonorrhœa, and is often the result of the empirical treatment of it by injections and cauterization—expedients which we can never too much condemn.

Strictures of the urethra cannot always be cured solely by the use of specifics. It would be impossible to destroy tissues which, although abnormal, are completely organized, and endowed with all the forces of vitality. We are therefore left to the necessity of reducing these newly formed structures by the aid of mechanical means. When this condition has been attained, the case comes into the category of traumatic inflammation, and consequently is amenable to medicinal forces. We immediately bring the specific action of Venereo into request as soon as the operation is finished—and it is only by such a course of treatment that good results can be expected; we repeat this operation twice a day, morning and evening, and at each occasion we inject cold water in which 20 or 25 globules of Venereo have been dissolved. Soon a purulent discharge will be set up, showing that inflammation has invaded the substance of the stricture, which attacked thus directly by the mechanical action of the bougie and the specific action of the Venereo, will soon yield and be destroyed. As a rule we have not merely one obstruction to overcome; and when the presence of others is ascertained, the same operation must be repeated on the second, then the third, and so on till all have been separately disposed of.

This operative treatment, effectively seconded by the employment of internal measures, and by injections of Venereo, will entirely clear the urethral canal of all kinds of obstructions.

The dietetic *régime* which must be pursued during the course of acute gonorrhœa, and even during the treatment of its chronic sequelæ, is exactly the opposite to that which must as a rule be followed in the case of syphilis, primary, constitutional or tertiary. Gonorrhœa is accompanied by an erysipelatous inflammation, which spreads widely over the mucous membrane, over which a quantity of capillary vessels and fine nervous twigs are dispersed. From this condition a state of vascular turgescence and reaction arises, which is felt in the whole cardiac and vascular system. Low diet, beverages of iced water, repose, and continued use of suspensory bandages, are here indispensable. In such cases, while we combat the essential blood disease by the external use of Venereo, we should at the same time promote atrophy of these fleshy formations by using a thread to constrict their base. After the fall of these excrescences external treatment must be continued, in order to anticipate and prevent the relapses which are so common in these cases.

THE LIQUID ELECTRICITIES AND THEIR APPLICATION.

The electricities are essential adjuncts in the treatment of disease. They are used both externally and internally, especially externally. The entire range of these valuable remedies is not even yet fully ascertained. Some recent discoveries, relating to their polarity and their co-relation with the physiological relations of electricity, as expounded by Dr. Chazarain and Dr. Décle, will be found in a subsequent chapter.

These liquids, a kind of electroids, are five in number.

I. *Red liquid, with electric properties, or Red Electricity.*—This has a positive action, and is suitable to lymphatic temperaments, in disorders of the stomach and abdomen, in nerve pains and sciatica, because the human body is generally electrically negative. If applied above and below the orbit, it strengthens sight.

II. *Yellow fluid, with electric properties, or Yellow Electricity.*—This has a negative action, and is efficacious when others fail. It is opposed in action to Red Electricity, and therefore neutralizes its exuberant effects. It is required when any excess of vital action is to be treated. It is also a vermifuge. The alternate use of Red and Yellow electricity are powerful agents in hastening convalescence.

III. *White fluid, with electric properties, or White Electricity.*—This is neutral in its action. It is especially used in the form of compresses on the head, and especially in affections of the abdomen. It is suitable to all constitutional types.

IV. *Blue fluid, with electric properties, or Blue or Angioitic Electricity.*—This has a positive action, and is used to control the blood-vessels. It acts also in varices, in hæmorrhages, and on all disease of the blood and blood-vessels. Taken internally in fifty-drop doses, it is a heroic remedy for apoplexy. It is the electricity for the sanguine type of temperament.

V. *Green fluid, with electric properties, or Green Electricity.*—This has a negative action. It is employed to promote cicatrization. It is especially useful in articular (or joint) pains and in cancer.

As a rule these liquids are employed externally, and sometimes, by means of injections, internally.

The various kinds of electricity have very different action, but are found to be equally powerful according to the temperament of the patient and the more or less pronounced development of the disease. This action is rapid, sometimes instantaneous. In rare cases it causes a shock similar to that produced by a small voltaic pile.

Eight or ten times only during twenty years, it has occurred to me to witness this singular phenomenon. But it must be observed that, as a rule, those who subject themselves to Electro-Homœopathic treatment do not take any pains to observe with accuracy the immediate effects of our specifics.

One of the most valuable, and at the same time most remarkable, effects of the electricities, is to relieve and very often entirely to remove pain without in any way disturbing the organism.

Certain diseases, when they do not arise from a very marked degeneration of the lymph or blood, are cured very rapidly, and sometimes even instantly, by simple applications of the electricity. In this way we have caused the immediate removal of partial tetanus by the application of Yellow Electricity to the occiput. Similarly, by using the appropriate electricity, we have cured innumerable cases of amaurosis, of chronic cephalalgia, rheumatism, sciatica, pains in the joints, and a case of stammering in a person forty-eight years of age.

Science has recognized the close correspondence between blood and nerves. Cures by the electricities alone—which act on the nerves—and, *per contra*, the removal of certain nervous diseases by means of remedies which purify the blood, are sufficient to give hourly proof how well grounded is this idea. Electricities, however, cannot, if used alone, cure a constitutional disease ; if a disorder of this nature has to be treated, internal treatment is indispensable. But even in these cases the electricities, as an adjunct, are a powerful auxiliary in hastening cure and, especially, in shortening convalescence.

As health results from—or is a resultant of—equilibrium established among all the vital forces, it is not to be denied that there is some truth in Brown's doctrine by which all disease is referred to either a sthenic or asthenic type—a condition of plus, or minus, strength. We become ill by either excess or defect of force; health is seated in the happy medium—the *via media* or *juste-milieu*. Accordingly we have found great advantage in the alternate use of Red and Yellow Electricity, especially during convalescence.

The extinction, or at least the relief, of pain is certainly a most conspicuous advantage which the electricities secure in a multitude of cases, especially in cancerous ulceration, and in wounds and lacerations of all kinds. The discovery of this inestimable resource for ameliorating suffering is surely a reason for thankfulness, and a motive for extending the knowledge of this therapeutic agent as widely as possible.

But it is especially in the treatment of scrofulous diseases that the use of the electricities to corroborate internal treatment is attended with the most remarkable results.

The electricities are used—

1. *As compresses:* A small piece of linen is moistened with a few drops, and applied directly to the painful part.

2. *By cupping:* That is by the application of the open mouth of the bottle containing the fluid to the cutaneous extremities of the nerves corresponding to the affected region, or over the suffering muscles.

Points of application.—The proper place to apply the electricities is generally indicated by the seat of pain, disease, or injury—contusions, wounds, lacerations, &c.

In all cases we should carefully select, as I have before observed, those places where the nerves are nearest the surface, or the place where pain is most felt. To assist the application of this rule, the plates at the end of this volume have been designed. To these we refer the reader who wishes to become thoroughly qualified to employ our system.

The following more definite suggestions may here be given. To act upon—

The whole body: Application should be made to the occiput, the great sympathetic centre, the solar plexus, the course of the dorsal spine, the points between the ribs on each side where the intercostal nerves come to the surface, and the soles of the feet.

The right side of the head: Apply the electricities to the right temple, to the forehead, above and below the orbit, and to the root of the nose.

The left side of the head: The corresponding points on the left side.

The tongue: To the greater and especially the lesser hypoglossal nerves.

The eyes: To the occiput, the great sympathetic, the supra and infra orbital regions.

The nose: To the root of the nose between the eyes; to the occiput, and above and below the orbit.

The ears: To the three small muscles behind the ear, but especially to the bases of the ear. And for this the mouth should be opened, and compresses of Red or White Electricity applied to the place where the ear touches the jaw. We may also use gargles of the positive electricities, but never of the Yellow or Green.

The arms: See the points indicated on the plate.

The legs: See the plate. Also touch the sacral nerves, and the sides of the dorsal spine and beneath the arch of the foot.

The bladder, the uterus, and adjacent parts: Apply the electricities to the sacral nerves, the perinæum, the pubes, and the great sympathetic.

Generally the seat of pain will sufficiently indicate what points should be touched; a little practice will soon render the use of the electricities easy.

Length of time for application.—If by *cupping*, the time varies from three to thirty seconds. Applications for seven, ten, or fifteen seconds are generally the most effectual. We advise short and often repeated applications. *Compresses* are left on till the linen is dry. They may be renewed more or less frequently, according to the effect obtained.

If pain has to be treated, we always begin by the use of one of the electricities; if pain returns, internal treatment must be superadded.

As a rule the Red Electricity is that which is first selected, most illness being the result of deficient vitality and therefore negative in type. The Red and Yellow are alternated in order to restore the neutral state of equilibrium, or health. These alternations, especially during convalescence, are very valuable. If pain is under treatment, we should wait for the effect of Red Electricity before passing on to Yellow. But if we wish to disperse any humours, or to act simply on the vital economy, the alternate use of Red and Yellow should be immediate.

When neither Red nor Yellow produce any effect, compresses of White Electricity should be used, especially for the head. This is always salutary. If neither of these three act, the reason must be that some degeneration of the blood or the lymph is present, for otherwise one of the three certainly would produce some effect.

Blue Electricity is applicable, as we have already remarked, to sanguine temperaments. We must not, however, be lax or heedless in the choice of electricities. We must in the first place ascertain decidedly whether the patient has a sanguine or lymphatic temperament, since experience has demonstrated that, in sanguine temperaments, the use of the Red and Yellow Electricities may give rise to disturbance, transient doubtless, but which it is better to avoid. Accordingly, with such patients we keep exclusively to the Blue or Angioitic Electricity. We can recognize the vigour of its action in the treatment of wounds. Good compresses disperse pain, stop hæmorrhage, and even bring together the divided surfaces of injured arteries.

In a case of wounded brachial arteries, an inexperienced medical attendant could not properly dress the wound, and the patient, after hæmorrhage lasting for eighteen hours, was at the point of death. Large compresses of Angioitic Electricity stopped the bleeding, and even closed the artery, and the man's life was saved. This might have seemed impossible if it had not actually occurred.

Green Electricity, applied by compresses, is especially serviceable in assuaging the pains of open cancer. It is used either undiluted, or added to water according to need, and according to the susceptibility of the patient. It may be used in all kinds of wounds; but in the relief of articular (joint) pains its effects are most triumphant. The doses must be adapted to particular cases.

Experience shows that prostration of vital force

is increased by the application of Yellow Electricity. Red Electricity, on the other hand, re-establishes force, sometimes even instantaneously, by simple contact with the injured part.

In a case of partial tetanus, caused by a wound, Yellow Electricity, applied to the occiput, to the great sympathetic, and to the wound itself, caused the immediate relaxation of the nerves, while Red Electricity had only increased the suffering.

Relying on observations such as these, which have been repeatedly renewed, I adopt the name of *Vegetable Electricity*, *positive* or *negative*.

In acute diseases these electricities, suitably selected, render great service. Thus in cases of severe erysipelas in the face, application of Red Electricity to the occiput, the great sympathetic, the forehead, above and below the orbit, caused the pain to disappear, and the inflammation and general pain ceased. In painful conditions of the nerves issuing between the ribs, in effusion in the chest, or pleurisy, electricity applied to the sympathetic and to the solar plexus, with the internal use of $Scrofoloso_1$ and $Pettorale_1$, dispel the fever, and allay the oppression, the pain, and all the gravest symptoms.

In acute sciatica, if we do not succeed by electricity applied to the sciatic and sacral nerves, we must employ unctions of $Canceroso_5$ and $Angioitico_2$, alternately.

In apoplexies we must, in the first place,

ascertain the cause in order to select with certainty the most appropriate electricity, for those which are suitable to nervous apoplexy are by no means adapted for sanguineous or hæmorrhagic cases.

It is easily seen, by what we have now said, how great is the influence of electricities, and how they may aid internal treatment. Thus in facial erysipelas we may see the diminution of the swelling almost as we are looking on. In ophthalmia, applications to the occiput, the sympathetic, the root of the nose, and the eyes, bring on the relief of lachrymation, while swelling and inflammation are reduced. In wounds, electricity immediately brings about effusion of humours and a crisis of suppuration.

In reference to the electricities the following particulars relative to the observations of Dr. Chazarain and Dr. Dècle, of Paris, may be added.

Dr. Chazarain and Dr. Dècle, of Paris, have discovered the polarity of man, that is to say, they have shown that one half of the human body is positive, and the other half negative.

And, after many laborious experiments, they have succeeded in pointing out, as is shown in the following table, which parts are positive, and which negative.

This discovery explains the intricacies of Animal Electricity, when applied empirically, and also the importance of positive and negative Vegetable

Electricity, which can be employed rationally and not empirically for the good of the sick.

Positive Electricity.	Negative Electricity.
RED.	YELLOW.
WHITE.	GREEN.*
BLUE.	

To employ the electricities, remove the cork from the bottle and apply the mouth of the bottle to the seat of the pain, for eight or ten seconds.

In rare cases these electricities give a shock.

The Positive and the Negative Electricity applied alternately to the pit of the stomach, to the solar plexus, to the occiput, to the centre of the cranium, to all the points of contact of the two electricities, give force to the whole body and to the voice. When applied to the little hypoglossi (see table at end of the book) they remove stammering, if care be taken to touch the right hypoglossal nerves with Red or Positive (+ Electricity), and the left hypoglossal with Yellow or Negative (— Electricity).

A toothache is cured by touching the jaw on the outside, over the seat of pain, with Yellow (negative) Electricity if the pain is on the left side, with Red Electricity (positive) if it is on the right.

* The names of colours by which the electricities are called are simply given for the sake of distinction, and not with the view of claiming the discovery of coloured electricities, as is alleged by certain persons who are interested in throwing ridicule on Count Mattei's great work.

Pains, confined to one side of the head (hemicrania), are cured by touching the nerve nearest to the little hypoglossal (see table); with Red or Positive Electricity if the pain is on the right side, and with Yellow or Negative, if it is on the left.

Erysipelas on the face will disappear if Red (positive) and Yellow (negative) Electricity be applied alternately to the occiput, and Red Electricity alone to the right super- and sub-orbital nerves, and Yellow Electricity to the left super- and sub-orbital nerves. Beginners should consult the tables at the end of the book in order to find the proper points to touch.

To remove deafness, apply the open bottle to the three muscles beneath the back of the ear, using Red Electricity for the right side, and Yellow Electricity for the left.

To treat semi-Anchylosis, touch those parts of the nerves which are nearest to the skin; thus, in the case of the knee, the nerves on the outer side must be touched with Yellow or Negative Electricity, those on the inner side with the Red or Positive Electricity, and the nerves above and beneath the knee with the positive and negative, alternately, as these are the points of contact of the two electricities.

The sight may be treated by touching the occiput with the Positive and Negative Electricities alternately, and by applying Red (positive) Electricity to the right super- and sub-orbital nerves, and Yellow (negative) to the corresponding nerves on the left.

For colds in the head (coryza) and chills, touch the root of the nose with the (positive) Red and (negative) Yellow Electricities, alternately.

In case of sciatica, touch the point where the sciatic nerve issues with Yellow (negative) Electricity, but the hollow of the foot with Red (positive) Electricity.

For a hemiplegia on the right side touch the occiput with the positive and negative Electricities alternately, the right side of the face with Red (positive) Electricity, the outer half of the arm and leg with Yellow (negative) and the inner half with Red (positive) Electricity.

Tic-douloureux on the left side of the face is removed by Yellow Electricity, on the right by Red Electricity.

Pains in the womb are removed by touching the sacral nerves (see table at the end) on the right side with Red Electricity (positive), and on the left with Yellow (negative), and on the ovaries with the Yellow and Red alternately.

Difficult childbirth may be assisted by touching the sacral nerves as above. The same treatment is applicable for hysteria.

The great sympathetic, which lies on each side of the atlas (see table), and is a most important nerve, owing to its ramifications in almost all the organs of the body, should be touched, as we have already mentioned, by the Yellow (negative) Electricity on the left side, and by the Red (positive) Electricity on the right.

To alleviate the pain of sores, wounds, bruises, or contusions, it is always best to touch the nerves which correspond with the painful spot, and the parts where the nerves are nearest the skin. If the wounds are on the inner side of the arm or leg, the Red (positive) Electricity should be used, if on the outside the Yellow (negative). If the wounds are on the right side of the thorax, the nerves must be touched with the Red (positive) Electricity, if on the left by the Yellow (negative).

Compresses may also be applied to the sores, wounds, or contusions, provided that the rule be followed of applying Positive Electricity to the negative parts, and, *vice versâ*, Negative Electricity to the positive parts.

DOSES AND METHOD OF APPLICATION OF THE GLOBULE REMEDIES.

We now propose giving general instructions for doses; but absolute rules cannot be given, since, from the infinite variety of organisms, numerous exceptions must arise. Thus a large field must be left to individual experience. The most common dose, for internal remedies, is one globule a day, in the first dilution. The second dilution is better in some cases, particularly with women and sensitive persons. Still, in certain cases, 10 to 20 dry globules of the remedy, which is being taken in solution, can be taken, or the same quantity may be taken of a second remedy, when they must be alternated with the remedy dissolved in water. The third dilution is given only where the disease assumes very violent forms, as in hysteria, epilepsy, typhus, &c.

Dilutions.—The *first dilution* is obtained by dissolving one globule in an ordinary glassful of water; we call it also the *first glass.*

To obtain the *second dilution*, a teaspoonful of the first dilution is put to a second glass of water. This is the *second glass.* The *third glass*, or the *third dilution*, is obtained in the same manner by taking a spoonful of the second preparation.

The remedy is taken by teaspoonfuls, so that the glassful may be finished during the day.

It must not be forgotten that the dose must be diminished according to the gravity or violence of the illness, and the smaller the doses, the closer must the intervals between them be, except in certain cases, which we shall indicate in the division of the book relating to the treatment of particular diseases.

External Use.—The globules are applied externally in different manners, viz., in *baths, compresses, unctions, gargles.*

To prepare an ordinary *bath* (of soft water), dissolve 100, 150, or 200 globules in a glass of water, and add it to the bath water.

For *compresses* and *gargles*, 20 to 25 globules must be melted in an ordinary glassful of water. For an *unction*, dissolve 5 globules in a drop of water, which must be mixed with a spoonful of oil, lard, or glycerine. The electricities are also used for baths and gargles. The proportion is 3 tablespoonfuls of electricity for a bath, and from 8 to 10 drops for a gargle. The compresses should be re-dipped three times a day, and even more often if it is found necessary. It is needless to remark that the external action of the globules is in no way different to their internal action.

The doses are increased in proportion as the disorder diminishes, for the simple reason that the remedies follow the law of similars and act homœopathically, and consequently reaction is decreased as the disease is subdued.

It is impossible to specify precisely all the circumstances which may require modification of the doses. It would be necessary to follow, step by step, the different phases of an infinite number of disorders which assume a thousand various aspects. It devolves upon the person who has the care of the patient to judge, from the state of the patient, what dose must be employed.

Nevertheless, we think it well to give here some rules derived from experience, and which should be carefully considered.

If a mistake is made in the choice of a remedy, no effect will be produced. If, on the contrary, aggravation is produced, it shows that the correct remedy is found; the dose must simply be diminished until no more aggravation is produced.

The effects of a remedy will be always immediate, provided that it is applied to a disorder included in its sphere of action. Consequently, if after several spoonfuls no result is produced, or if, in spite of the diminution of the dose, aggravation continues, the conclusion may be drawn that the remedy is not suitable to the disease under treatment. The aggravation is always only transient, and is in no way dangerous.

But, whether in diminishing the dose, in turning to the homologies or varieties of the remedy, or in changing the remedy altogether, success is always certain.

These modifications must be learnt by trial, by preliminary courses of experience, which will soon lead to habits of precision.

Small doses do not lessen the action of the remedy; they put it *en rapport* with the state of the patient.

In the case of infants the remedy may be given to the nurse; for young children the second dilution is given.

The necessity of taking the remedies in low dilutions, and of repeating the spoonfuls frequently in grave cases, is explained by the fact that the remedies have an instantaneous action, terminating immediately after their absorption; hence they must be often repeated in order to secure good results. And experience has shown that when too much is taken, the overplus is inoperative.

The remedy must be taken up to the time of meals, and even during meal-time.

There is no reason why the remedies should not be given during menstruation: it is, on the contrary, a good time, as the blood is then more active in expelling morbid principles.

Only it must be noted that the Angioitics, in ordinary doses, bring back the suppressed periodic flux, while in small doses they are specific for opposite conditions of menorrhagia, or excessive flow, and for hæmorrhages generally.

The only diet required is that which supplies healthy and sufficient nourishment. Strong acids, such as vinegar and lemons, are antidotes to our remedies. The remedies are never mixed. Compresses and unctions of two different remedies must be given in succession, not in combination Also, when in complicated disorders several remedies are used, they must be given separately and successively, taking care to alternate them.

Seeing that the action of each spoonful is of short duration, it is not absolutely necessary to set apart a certain portion of the day to each of the two remedies; they can be also alternated in doses, *i.e.*, by taking a spoonful of the first, and then soon afterwards a spoonful of the second, and so on, at prescribed intervals.

The water for the compresses or baths, or for internal use, may be cold, tepid, more or less hot, according to taste. It can also be sweetened with sugar.

PRACTICAL RÉSUMÉ.

The following summary of the chief modes of using the Electro-Homœopathic remedies may be found useful.

1. The first dilution is prepared by dissolving one globule in an ordinary tumblerful of drinking water—or better distilled water. It is advisable to use a glass of about the same measure in preparing the subsequent dilutions.

2. The second dilution is obtained by adding a teaspoonful of the first dilution to a second glassful of water.

The dilutions are often indicated by Roman numerals following the sign of the medicine. Thus SI, SII, means the first and second dilution of Scrofoloso.

3. Remedies so prepared are taken by teaspoonful doses about every 10 or 15 minutes, according to the gravity of the case, so as to finish the prescribed quantity during the day.

4. Medicine may be taken immediately before and after a meal as well as during the intervals.

5. Some globules of the medicine taken in dilution may be also taken, at each meal, in a little wine or water.

6. When two medicines are prescribed simultaneously, one should be taken in the morning, the other in the afternoon, half a glassful of each. In this case, the globules for meal-times should be taken as follows: at breakfast-time, some globules of the medicine taken in dilution during the morning; and at dinner, globules of the medicine taken in dilution during the afternoon.

7. Patients who are unable to take remedies in dilution may take the globules dry, every half-hour or hour.

8. When several dry globules are prescribed, the given number is placed on the tongue, and left to dissolve gradually.

9. The electricities may be taken internally, a few drops for a dose, once a day or oftener, either in a little water or on sugar.

10. Treatment need not be discontinued during the monthly illness.

11. Nursing infants may be treated by medicine given to the nurse; young children should have the medicines in the second dilution or dry globules.

12. The only rule for diet is to take wholesome and sufficient food. In grave cases acids, such as vinegar and lemon-juice, should be avoided.

EXTERNAL APPLICATIONS.

13. *For Baths.* — Dissolve 100, 150, or 200 globules in a glassful of warm water, and stir this into the bath. Patients may remain in the bath

15 to 20 minutes, or longer, if the bath is agreeable as well as salutary. Baths may also be medicated by the electricities ; a tablespoonful (or a bottleful) for each bath.

14. *Gargles, Compresses, Injections, Enemas.*—Twenty globules in a glass of warm or cold water. Compresses should be renewed as often as necessary to keep them fresh.

For gargling with the electricities, the dose is 8 or 10 drops to a tumblerful of water.

15. *Unctions.*—Dissolve 5 crushed globules in a drop of water and add a tablespoonful of oil, or of glycerine, and mix thoroughly. Take a little of this preparation in the hollow of the hand and rub it gently on the parts indicated.

16. *Lotions* are prepared by dissolving 20 globules in a teaspoonful of water and mixing this with a tablespoonful of spirits of wine. In using this, take up by a sponge a few drops of the lotion, or apply it by a camel's-hair brush to the scalp or face. It may be applied to other parts by a small piece of flannel.

17. *The Electricities* are either used pure, by cupping, *i.e.*, inverting the open bottle, applied to the affected part; or they may be mixed with water, a teaspoonful to a tumblerful of water, and used as compresses.

Instead of the cupping process, the electricities may be applied by a camel's-hair brush, or by the hollow of the hand, as directed for the unctions.

18. When two electricities are prescribed alternately, the second may be applied after a short interval—that is to say, as soon as the first is dry. These applications may be repeated night and morning, or, in acute and neuralgic cases, as often as may be necessary.

Such are the rules by which any one who can distinguish between a lymphatic and a sanguine subject can suitably administer the remedies. We could give many examples proving that an error in the choice of a remedy or dose can indefinitely retard the cure of a disorder.

One woman, amongst others, having a cancer in the breast and being subject to hæmorrhage, the hæmorrhage was very much increased by putting two globules in the glass instead of one. This aggravation ceased when the mistake was corrected and she returned to the prescribed dose. Impatient to be cured, she again doubled the dose, but the hæmorrhage this time assumed alarming proportions; then again it disappeared under the action of Angioitico and Canceroso in ordinary doses.

If the state of the patient is grave, it is prudent always to commence with the second dilution, reserving an increased dose till later on.

There are cases in which the very smallest doses, the third dilution for example, are necessary, as in organic diseases of the heart, epilepsy, hysteria, and convulsive disorders in general.

In other cases, strong doses must be employed without hesitation; twenty to thirty globules dry on the tongue, at the commencement of cholera, generally stop it; in asphyxia, the same results are obtained by a similar process.

Finally, there are persons who find it better to take eight or ten globules dry, one every hour, instead of the dilution. These are special cases, which are explained by differences of organization, and which must be left to individual observation. But in serious diseases, it is of great importance to keep to the prescribed doses.

One of the numerous advantages which Electro-Homœopathy gives us is that of being able to act immediately should there be doubts of the results of the diagnosis. Scrofoloso 1 and 5, administered in an ordinary dose, will certainly lead to amelioration if the disease is in their sphere of action; if not, they will put the practician on the right track by arousing symptoms which will leave no doubt as to the type of the disease.

It is especially in diseases of the liver and spleen—in disease arising from intestinal worms, especially tænia—that hesitation may arise, and in which a wrong decision may be dangerous.

There is nothing more capricious than these diseases; the doctors make mistakes in them as well as the most ignorant of amateurs. In the last-named cases, Vermifugo and the new Febrifugo will be the touchstones which will speedily reveal the nature of the disease.

The obstinacy of certain disorders is sometimes due to hereditary syphilitic taint. When the diagnosis is doubtful, Venereo should be alternated with the appropriate specific. This must not be neglected, particularly in certain cases of cancer, scirrhus, suspicious wounds, never forgetting, however, that $Canceroso_1$ is also specific for inveterate syphilitic virus.

No one can deny that the new therapeusis has passed the bounds laid down by allopathy; every disease which is regarded as incurable succumbs, sooner or later, to our remedies.

It is a great advance; and we are assured that our science has not yet spoken its last word. But it is a great fact which we can affirm, without fear of contradiction, that a dead body can be electrified but can never be resuscitated. Thus we may meet with a case in which the whole mass of the blood is entirely corrupt, and the different functions completely disorganized. We can certainly give relief, we can for a time confer a sort of artificial life, but a cure in such a case is impossible; our powers cannot go beyond the limits of finite human force. We can only say that every disease must be *taken in time.*

EASY EXPERIMENTS.

Many persons have heard of Electro-Homœopathy; others have read or will read books on the subject; but as there are persons—the majority, perhaps—who must be dealt with not so much with arguments which persuade as by facts which compel, who are only accessible to the coarsest and most obstinate of arguments—we will here indicate the means of making easy experiments which require no medical knowledge.

1. Eight or ten globules of Scrofoloso dry will render an intoxicated man sober, will stop a threatening of paralysis, or arrest an attack of fainting, &c.

2. Two or three globules of the same remedy on the tongue will restore digestion if it is difficult or arrested, or give appetite and sleep; stop cramp of the stomach, allay toothache, &c.

3. Several spoonfuls of Canceroso, of the first or second dilution, often immediately stop spasmodic contractions of the womb; and by means of this remedy sufficiently continued, all the ailments which trouble a woman during and after confinement can be stopped.

4. Strong compresses of Angioitic Electricity stop the pain and arrest the flow of blood from a wound, and make it speedily close and heal.

5. Several compresses of White Electricity stop immediately neuralgia in the head; one gargle is often sufficient to stop the most obstinate toothache.

6. A sufficiently prolonged treatment with Scrofoloso, and applications of Red Electricity will cause

the solution and expulsion of a calculus, the closure of a hernia, and will bring back colour and life to chlorotic patients.

7. Fevers and liver diseases may be stamped out by Febrifugo, internally, and unctions of Febrifugo novo.

These are experiments which beginners may make in order to prove the surprising efficacy of the Electro-Homœopathic medicines.

It is very generally supposed that confidence or faith is necessary in order to feel the good effects of the remedies; allopaths say that this is the secret of homœopathy. It cannot be said with regard to medicine that faith suffices. Can it be faith or confidence which cures the suckling infant who has no other medicines but those which are given through the nurse? What faith can an intoxicated man, a person in a fainting fit, a madman, have, who are nevertheless cured? Doubtless confidence is necessary, but not that the effect of the remedy may be obtained, but that the prescribed course may be carried out with sincerity and intelligence. Faith is also necessary especially for beginners, in order to induce them not to put too many globules in the glass, seeing they are so small; there must be confidence that the patient may persevere for the time necessary to secure the result, to avoid the temptation to grasp after a more rapid cure by the use of stronger doses. Confidence is only necessary at the commencement; once the results are seen, conviction and certainty follow.

ANATOMICAL AND PHYSIOLOGICAL PRINCIPLES.

In order that persons unacquainted with medicine may derive profit from our instructions, and to make the study of an experimental materia medica more easy for them, we have judged it well to give several anatomical and physiological data, which, though contained within a few pages, will suffice, we believe, to explain the structure of the human body, and the different functions of our organs, in respect to that which concerns the vegetative and the higher spheres of life. The human body, which, from a mechanical point of view, is a very perfect and complex structure, is nevertheless of such a simple nature that in no other machine can its like be found, however great may be the genius which has contrived it. Everything is found here: models of levers, pulleys of all kinds, joints of all forms; art has never been able to construct in optics any apparatus as complete as the eye; in music, nothing so varied and perfect as the voice, the hearing, &c.

Man is a master-piece, the plan of which God only could have conceived, and in which ever increasing and profound study is constantly discovering new and marvellous details. His organs, admirably distributed, are composed of solids and liquids.

The solid organs are the bones, cartilage, muscles, tendons, aponeuroses or sheaths, nerves, viscera, &c.

For liquids there are the blood, the chyle, the bile, sweat, urine, saliva, tears, &c.

The bones represent the framework of the human body; hard, solid, and resisting, at once forming resting-places or platforms for the other organs, sometimes cavities to protect them; and the outward form is always modelled upon them. Completely passive, they only share in movement when called upon by muscular action. The difference in form which is observed in the bones, has suggested a division of them into long, short, and flat bones.

The first are found where large movement is required, as, for example, in the limbs; short bones are found in parts which are required to possess at once great flexibility and great solidity, as, for example, in the hand, the foot, the vertebral column. Flat bones, those in which length and width predominate over thickness, are generally used to form protective cavities for the organs; they are found in the head, the chest, and the pelvis.

The structure of the bones varies according to their form and position, and is always found to correspond to their use, consequently, in the long bones which require much solidity, compact tissue predominates, whilst the cellulous or spongy substance predominates in short bones,

The bones are surrounded by a thin, solid, and adhering membrane, which follows the nutritious blood-vessels into the interior of the organ, and is called the periosteum.

Muscles are organs formed by the long parallel, red or reddish, and contractile fibres; they are intended to supply movement to the different parts of the body; they are joined to the bones at their points of attachment by means of tendons and sheaths, which are almost rounded or membranous prolongations of the periosteum.

The human body, which is for the most part symmetrically constructed, consists of the trunk and the limbs. The trunk is the central or principal part, which contains the most vital organs and the viscera. It consists of three cavities—the head, the chest, and the abdomen.

The head contains the centre of the nervous system, the brain, and the principal organs of the senses.

The chest, united to the head by means of the neck, contains the respiratory and circulatory organs; the posterior region is called the back, and the anterior acts as a support to the breasts, the lactiferous organs.

The diaphragm, a very strong muscle, separates the chest from the abdomen.

The abdomen contains the organs of digestion, of secretion, excretion, and generation.

To facilitate the study of the parts contained in the abdomen, it must be looked upon as divided into three great enclosures or belts, by means of two imaginary horizontal lines, and two other vertical ones, thus producing nine regions. The middle region of the upper belt is called the epigastrium; the two side ones are the hypochondria. The middle region of the central belt is the umbilical region, the side ones the lumbar divisions; finally, the middle region of the lower belt has been called the hypogastrium, and the side regions the iliac fossæ. The posterior of the abdomen takes the name of the loins; the folds separating the stomach from the thighs is called the groin. The limbs, articulated appendages intended for movement, are divided into superior, thoracic, or pectoral limbs, and inferior, pelvic, or abdominal limbs.

The articulations divide all these several limbs into many parts, viz.: the shoulders, arms, forearms, and the hands, ending in the fingers or upper limbs; the thigh, ending at one end in the hips and the other in the knee; the leg, the foot ending in the toes and heel, or lower limbs.

The nervous system is composed of a large number of filaments, called nerves, and is completed by the co-aptation of various organs and apparatus, by means of which communication is carried on between the organs of the body and the outward world. This system is composed of a soft and pulpy substance which is almost liquid in its primitive state, and acquires a firmer consistency as age advances.

This substance, called nervous tissue, is very variable in its aspect; it is white, or grey, or ash-coloured; sometimes it forms more or less bulky masses, and sometimes long and ramifying cords; these last organs are called nerves, and the first, ganglions or nervous centres, because they gather all the nerves into one system.

The common centre, known by the name of the medulla oblongata, is formed by the central extremities of the nerves and by several fibres which compose the hemispheres of the brain and the cerebellum. These, united, form the brain or cerebrum in the head.

Besides, this centre is very largely constituted by the spinal cord, which, extended into the vertebral column, seems to be composed simply of filaments continuous with the nerves, and which originate in it. It is then easily understood that the function of the nerves is to establish harmony and relation amongst all the organs of the human body.

The hemispheres of the brain are formed by the separate medullary fibres, extended into the grey substance, in which they cross one with another and amalgamate. These internal or central nervous tissues have a very complicated structure.

The cerebellum is the resultant of the smaller separate spinal fossæ which constitute the spinal cord. These form a number of little plates, so divided by the ash-coloured substance which crosses them, that they are very analogous to a Voltaic pile.

There are several subordinate apparatus which add to the perfection of the nervous system; they are composed of nerves having special functions—that is to say, they carry to a common sensorium the impressions made by outward objects. The peripheric extremities are supplied with organs suitable to receive these impressions. These organs, called senses, are constructed in accordance with the physical laws which are adapted to excite them, as is seen in the structure of the eye, the ear, the nostrils, and the tongue.

The nerves branching into these organs are the olfactory nerves, the optic nerves, acoustic nerves, and those of taste, to which must be added the pneumo-gastric nerves which convey sensation of physical anxiety and hunger. The other nerves recognize the qualities of bodies which appeal to touch. The numerous and various phenomena which occur in our body always result from the correlated action of one or more parts of the body, and these parts, which may be considered as the principal instruments, are called organs. The combination of several organs for the production of the same phenomena form an organic system, and the action of an organ or system is called its function. In such a complicated machine as the human body, composed of so many organs, there must necessarily be a great many functions. Each individual having in the course of his existence two distinct missions to fulfil, that of individual preservation, and the preservation of the race, it is easy to recognize two classes of functions—those belonging to the individual life, and those concerned with the preservation of the race.

Functions of the first class may be divided, first, into functions entirely vegetative, by means of which the individual assimilates to its own substance the food with which it is nourished—that is to say, the functions of nutrition; secondly, the functions by means of which the individual is put *en rapport* with other individuals around it—that is to say, functions of relation.

The functions of nutrition include digestion, absorption, respiration, circulation, nutrition, and secretion. The functions of relation are the senses, voice, speech, and movement.

The functions of the second class, which secure the perpetuity of the race, are divided into generation, gestation, accouchement, and lactation.

DIGESTION.

Digestion is a function common to all animals, by means of which foreign substances introduced into the body, and subjected to the action of a particular system of organs, change their quality, and furnish a new composition which is suitable to their nourishment and growth.

Executed by a very complicated apparatus, digestion comprises many phenomena which it will be well to examine separately. These phenomena are: the ingestion of aliment or food, mastication, insalivation, deglutition or swallowing, chymification, chylification, absorption, and defecation.

The digestive tube, which, commencing at the mouth, ends in the anus, offers in its course a great number of parts, which, each in its own way, works for the same result.

The mouth is the first. The buccal cavity is limited above by the palate, below by the lower jaw, behind by the soft palate and the pharynx, in front by the teeth and lips, at the sides by the cheeks; in the middle is the tongue, which moves in every direction.

One of the two jaws, the lower one, is extremely movable, being governed by very powerful muscles; the other, the upper one, is completely immovable. Each jaw is provided, in the adult, with sixteen teeth, which are divided into two parts, the outer or exposed portion called the crown, and the inner or concealed portion called the root.

The mouth shows, also, on examination, the salivary glands, situated in the interior of the cheeks, at the junction of the lips and gums, and principally the two parotids, which meet beneath the skin between the eye and the jaw, and which open on to the mouth by means of a duct which crosses the cheek; the two submaxillary glands, situated in the central part of the lower jaw, and whose ducts open near the frœnum of the tongue.

If we examine the interior of an open mouth, with the tongue depressed, in the upper and back parts will be seen a transverse movable sort of partition, which is called the soft palate, which separates the mouth from the pharynx, and of which there is a prolongation called the uvula. On each side the arches of the palate are terminated in prolongations which are continuous with the tongue and pharynx, and in the middle of which are the tonsils. In the posterior part of the cavity, behind the soft palate, we see the opening of the pharynx, a membranous funnel-shaped canal, which is continuous with the œsophagus, a muscular membranous conduit, whose function it is to convey the food through the pharynx into the stomach.

The stomach, the principal organ of digestion, placed in a transverse position across the epigastric region, besides its cavity, has two openings. The one called the cardiac, the left, or the œsophageal orifice, where the gullet terminates, is found at a point defined by dividing the superior surface into three parts; the œsophageal opening is at the first division from the left side. The other, the pyloric or intestinal orifice, is below, somewhat anterior to the cardiac orifice, and to the right; it commences by a funnel-shaped enlargement, and ends abruptly in a circular contraction, around in the interior of which is found a little circular elevation called the pyloric sphincter.

The stomach consists of three coats, an exterior or serous coat, a middle or muscular coat, and an interior or mucous coat; and receives a great number of vessels and nerves. The intestines are the continuation of the stomach, and of smaller calibre, and divided into large and small intestines. The small intestines are the duodenum, the jejunum, and the ileum. The large intestine or colon, wider but shorter than the preceding, leads to the cæcum, the rectum, and the anal termination. The whole intestinal mass is covered by the omentum and invested with the peritoneum. The liver, the organ which secretes bile, assists in blood formation, and gives its characteristic products to the blood. It is the largest viscus in the body, and is placed in the upper right side of the abdomen, and extends as far as the level of the lower boundary of the ribs. Its upper surface is convex, and the lower irregularly concave; its colour a reddish brown. It is composed of a tender and compact substance, and if torn, it seems to be formed by the agglomeration of little lobules where the blood-vessels meet, where originate the ducts which convey the bile to the structures outside.

These biliary or gall ducts unite together, forming little branches, and afterwards, a trunk coming from the lower surface of the liver, reaches the duodenum, and also communicates with a membranous bag attached to the liver, nearly always filled with bile, and which is called the gall bladder.

The terminal duct discharges itself into the duodenum near the stomach.

The pancreas, which secretes the pancreatic juice, by which fatty substances are resolved into an emulsion, is a gland analogous to the salivary glands, a granular mass divided into several lobes, which sub-divide themselves into secondary ones.

The pancreas is tolerably compact, of a whitish-grey colour inclining to red; it is placed transversely between the stomach and the vertebral column. Each of the lobes composing this gland gives rise to a small duct, and all these ducts unite to form a canal which empties itself into the duodenum, near the mouth of that coming from the liver.

The spleen, a spongy viscus, of a ruddy pale-blue colour, also contributes to the formation of the bile, and is placed at the base of the left hypochondria, between the ventricle of the stomach and the vertebral ends of the ribs. It is of the shape of an egg cut lengthwise, and is formed by a somewhat thin vascular tissue enveloped in two membranes.

The absence of any excretory duct has made physiologists uncertain as to the use of this organ. However, it seems that the capillary tissue not only prepares the blood to receive the biliary secretion, but it supplies blood in large quantities to the short vessels when it is compressed by the stomach.

INGESTION OF FOOD, MASTICATION, AND INSALIVATION.

Food is conveyed by the hand to the mouth, and is immediately subjected to the grinding and masticating action of the teeth. The act of mastication, though very simple, involves the co-operation of the cheeks and tongue to collect the material, and to bring it repeatedly under the action of the jaws. During this time the salivary glands on each side, excited by the presence of food, secrete and pour out a large quantity of saliva.

In turn, when the grinding is completed, the tongue forms the whole collection into a rounded mass, and making an inclined passage, carries it forward to the throat. Then the veil of the palate rises and becomes horizontal to shut off the orifice of the nasal fossæ; the epiglottis is lowered to close the larynx, the larynx becomes elongated, and the food, pushed by an alternately partial dilating and contracting movement, descends through the œsophagus to the stomach. Deglutition is thus completed.

CHYMIFICATION, CHYLIFACTION, AND DEFECATION.

One of the most important phenomena of digestion takes place in the stomach. The elaboration to which the food is subjected in this organ is attributed to the action of a particular fluid, the gastric juice, secreted by the glands located in the walls of the stomach. After a shorter or longer space of time, the food is changed to a sort of liquid paste, of a grey colour, which is called chyme, and which, in proportion to its transformation, is carried towards the pylorus, which allows it to pass on to the duodenum, while it arrests those parts which are insufficiently digested. Sometimes, under the influence of different causes, the action of the stomach is reversed: it contracts violently, overcomes the resistance of the œsophagus, and, aided by the contractions of the abdominal muscles, throws out the matters which it contained. This is called vomiting.

Arrived in the duodenum, the chyme is mixed with the bile and pancreatic juice. The exact action of these liquids is unknown, but it is certain that they are indispensable to digestion. In any case, the chyme is modified, and a whitish alkaline liquid separates itself from it, called chyle, and which is absorbed by the multitudinous chyliferous vessels which open on to the internal surface of the intestine, whose function it is to absorb the essential part of the partially digested mass. In proportion as it advances through the slight peristaltic undulations of the small intestines, more and more of the nutritive mass is separated, until finally it arrives at the cæcum, whence it cannot return, being kept back by a muscular ring which acts as a valve and separates the ileum from the colon.

Here the digestive residuum is deposited and shaped, the remaining nutritive portions are taken, and when they have accumulated in sufficient quantity in the rectum, the need of ejecting them is felt ; the intestine contracts, and, aided by the combined efforts of the diaphragm and the muscles of the stomach, empties itself, and this constitutes the act of defecation. This is the history of human digestion.

ABSORPTION.

Absorption is the function by means of which living beings extract, through certain vessels, the elements useful for their sustenance. This act is exercised in the interior of our organs, in the digestive canal, on food and drink, and on the surface of our body by means of the integuments.

Whilst in certain animals absorption is only carried on by means of blood-vessels, in man, as well as in other animals with an equally complicated organization, it is effected by means of a system of canals called lymphatic vessels. These are little canals, beginning in very fine and small capillaries in the substance of the different organs, and which, after being united in a more or less voluminous trunk, empty themselves into the veins. They have very thin and transparent walls, and exist in all parts of the body. The greater number are collected into a large trunk called the thoracic duct. In their course, the lymphatic vessels cross the little round organs placed at the groins, the arm-pits, in the neck, chest, and abdomen.

The use and structure of these bodies, called lymphatic ganglions, are not yet well understood.

To render the study of the digestion easier, it is useful to know how the nutritive substance proceeding from the food passes from the stomach and intestinal tube into the mass of blood which it replenishes.

Several liquids and some of the solids introduced into the stomach are immediately absorbed by the veins, which form a network on the walls of this organ and of the small intestines; but the larger part of the fibrine and the fatty substances constituting the chyle take another route, and reach a special system of canals belonging to the apparatus of the lymphatic vessels, which, owing to the milky aspect which they present when they are distended by the chyle, also take the name of chyliferous vessels.

These originate on the surface of the intestinal mucous membrane, inosculate by a more or less crowded network spread between the two surfaces of the mesentery, pass through the mesenteric ganglions, and terminate in the thoracic duct which empties itself into the left subclavian vein.

RESPIRATION.

Respiration is the function by which air is introduced into a special organ to undergo decomposition, and to give to the fluids circulating through this organ one of the principles which enables them to vitalize the tissues.

Atmospheric air is the principal agent of respiration; and its organs are the trachea, the bronchi, and the lungs.

The trachea is a fibro-cartilaginous cylinder, placed in front of the vertebral column, acting as a conduit to the larynx, and which branches in the lower part and gives rise to two other conduits, which pass into the lungs. These conduits are the bronchi, which are divided into right and left; the right is wider, shorter, and more horizontal than the left.

On reaching the lung these two conduits divide into two other branches, which again divide and, after a short space, give rise to other smaller ramifications, the calibre of which diminishes as the branches multiply. They extend in all directions, and it is difficult to trace them to their terminations.

The trachea and the bronchi are composed of rings which, incomplete behind, are connected together by a solid membrane. Their interior surface is covered by a mucous membrane.

The lungs are two spongy, shiny organs, divided into a certain number of cells, into which the air penetrates, and on the walls of which the vessels ramify which contain the blood to be subjected to the influence of the oxygen contained in the atmosphere. They are placed in the chest, and are separated from one another by the heart and the mediastinum; they are called the right and the left lung. They are pale fawn in colour, approximating to white or grey. Their shape is difficult to define. The right is divided into three lobes, the left into two only. The exterior surface of both is polished and convex, and in direct contact with the walls of the chest; but, in a normal state, without any adhesion. The interior surface is flat or slightly concave. Near the centre is found the insertion of the bronchi. The lungs are each enclosed in the pleura, thin diaphanous membranes covering the interior of each side of the chest, and thence reflected over each lung. Their internal surfaces, as in all serous membranes, to which class they belong, always touch one another, and each is therefore a shut cavity.

They resemble two C's, which would touch one another in their convexities, thus: ƆC.

They form in the middle of the chest two triangular spaces, called mediastinæ, quite distinct from one another—anterior and posterior.

The respiration, the organs of which we have now described, takes place by means of two alternating movements of expansion and contraction of the chest-walls, called inspiration and expiration. These movements can only be properly effected under a certain atmospheric pressure, and when the air is composed of 21 parts of oxygen, 79 of nitrogen, and a small quantity of carbonic acid.

Animal heat, which is generally about 98° Fahr., seems to depend for the most part on the decomposition of the air during the act of respiration, which Lavoisier considered a true case of combustion. We can, at will, accelerate or slacken these respiratory movements, but we cannot suspend them entirely.

Inspiration, or the introduction of air into the lungs, takes place in the following manner: The diaphragm, which is an arch with the convexity upwards, contracts; the flat part becomes horizontal and pushes down the abdominal viscera; on the other side, the ribs, being acted upon by the muscles of respiration, rise, and at the same time yield to expansion of the chest.

In consequence of these movements the thorax enlarges, and the lungs increase in volume; the air is introduced through the mouth and the nose, passes along the larynx, the trachea, and the bronchial tubes, is sent through all its ramifications, and dilates the pulmonary air cells, whence it is finally expelled by expiration, after remaining for several seconds in the smallest air cells.

The quantity of air breathed in each inspiration

has been estimated at 30 to 40 cubic inches, but its composition, when analyzed on emerging from the lungs, is considerably changed, for, instead of 21 parts of oxygen and 79 of nitrogen, it only contains 0.14 of oxygen and 79 of nitrogen, but is charged with carbonic acid.

This change occurs from the contact of the air with the venous blood, which, in taking up the oxygen, turns from a dark colour to red, and is capable of supporting the life of the organs to which it is distributed.

Expiration, of which we have not yet spoken, takes place through a diametrically opposite mechanism to that of inspiration; that is to say, the diaphragm is loosened at the same time that the inspiratory muscles of the chest are contracted.

The organs of respiration also take part in certain phenomena which are continually taking place, such as laughing, coughing, sneezing, yawning, sighing, and sobbing.

Laughing, which generally shows itself when we hear or see anything pleasant and agreeable, is a succession of rapid, short inspirations, which draw in and cast out the air with a special sound, and varying with different people.

Coughing, always caused by an irritation of the respiratory canals, consists in a strong expiration, which clears the bronchial tubes and the trachea, and sends forth the matters constituting the sputa with a noise which constantly varies but is always recognizable.

Sneezing has some affinity with coughing, but with this difference, that it is always less frequent, and occasioned by an irritation of the nasal mucous membrane.

Yawning is a long inspiration, accompanied by a large opening of the jaws; one yawns for ennui, or when sleepy, or on waking, and it seems that in every case this phenomenon is for the purpose of rousing the enfeebled respiratory apparatus, or to raise the muscles of the thorax to the degree necessary for respiration, which is always more active during the waking hours than during sleep.

Sighing is of a similar nature, and occurs when the individual is much pre-occupied and forgets to breathe regularly. Owing to this want of continuous attention to respiration, it is necessary that from time to time a deep respiration should be made in order to dilate the extremest air cells.

Finally, sobbing consists in a spasmodic contraction of the diaphragm, which, causing the air to enter in a jerky, interrupted way, produces several hard, sonorous, and fatiguing inspirations.

CIRCULATION.

Circulation is the movement by which the blood, on leaving the heart, is carried continuously through all parts of the body, and which, through the medium of the veins, returns to the centre whence it started, after traversing the lungs in which it regains, by its contact with the air, those nutritive properties which it had lost in its passage through the organs. The instruments of this important function, which is entirely independent of the will, and necessarily connected with the respiration in the adult, are the heart, arteries, and veins.

The heart is a muscular organ, about the size of one's fist, irregularly conical with the base turned upwards, placed in the middle and anterior part of the chest, and a little to the left, between the two lungs, in the anterior mediastinum and surrounded by a serous bag called the pericardium.

The heart shows, on examination, two halves separated by a superficial cross groove and four cavities; two of these are in the body of the organ itself, and are called left and right ventricle; the other two, in the shape of appendices, communicate with the ventricles, and are called left and right auricles.

The communications between the auricles and ventricles are furnished with valves, that on the left being called the mitral valve, and that on the right the tricuspid valve.

The arteries are cylindrical vessels which convey the blood from the heart to all parts of the body. The walls of these vessels are thick and solid, and are composed of three membranes. From their final ramifications the arteries communicate with the veins by means of extremely thin divisions, which are called capillary vessels.

The veins, the structure and appearance of which differs from that of the arteries, receive the residue of the blood distributed through the arteries, and re-conducts it to the heart. The membranes of the veins are also three in number, but of a less consistency than those of the arteries; the interior contains several valves ordinarily placed near the branches, which prevents the blood from being carried back by the force of gravity.

As demonstrated by Harvey in the seventeenth century, the phenomena of circulation can be easily understood, in spite of its apparent complexity. We will explain it in a few words, and, in order to follow the circulation of the blood with greater ease, we will explain it from the moment when, collected from all the veins of the body, it flows into the vena-cava.

These veins, into which all the others empty themselves, turn the blood into the right auricle of the heart, which dilates to receive it, afterwards contracting to expel it into the ventricle of the same side.

Borne by these vessels into the lung, the blood is distributed through the ramifications of the artery to all the points of the respiratory organ, and comes into contact with the atmospheric air. It then absorbs oxygen, and by its combination with this gas is changed from black to red, and is introduced into the pulmonary veins, which re-conduct it into the left auricle of the heart. This receives the oxygenated blood, contracts, and passes it through the left ventricle, which, in turn, expels it into the aorta and thence to the whole arterial system.

The diastole, a dilating movement in the cavities of the heart, and the systole, a contracting movement, takes place at the same time in the two ventricles and in the two auricles, in such a manner that the diastole of the auricles corresponds in time with the systole of the ventricles and *vice versâ.*

These alternate movements constitute the beating of the heart, always accelerated by mental emotions, running, and by all muscular effort.

During the systole, the apex of the heart strikes the wall of the chest.

Pushed by the left ventricle, the arterial blood, or, to use a better term, the oxygenated blood, passes into the aorta, and thence is spread through all the organs by means of the arteries resulting from the innumerable divisions and subdivisions which are found in all parts of the body.

This liquid is made to flow by the impulse which the heart gives to it, and also by a kind of contractility inherent in the structure of the coats of the arteries.

The pulse is the undulating movement produced

in each artery; it reflects accurately the frequency and force of the beatings of the heart, and consequently the state of the circulation.

In the adult individual and in health the pulse is from sixty to seventy a minute, is quicker in children, and generally in women. After a certain number of subdivisions, the artery degenerates into many very small vessels which are called capillaries.

The blood penetrates by the means of these vessels through all our organs to deposit its nutritive elements; the capillaries take up this impoverished fluid, and it is borne by the veins to the heart, again to be submitted to the influence of the air in the lungs.

Then the heart is the centre of impulsion; the arteries carry the blood from the centre to the circumference, and the veins bring it back again to the centre.

SECRETIONS.

Secretion is the result of the elaboration of the blood in the organs specially constructed to appropriate certain portions and form out of it new products. Secretions may be classified as organic, excremental, and functional, according to their use and destination—whether they are intended to remain in the system to serve different purposes, or to be completely or partially rejected.

Physiology recognizes three kinds of secreting organs, viz., exhaling vessels, follicles, and glands.

The exhaling vessels are composed of small tubes which draw humour from the arteries to distribute it over certain surfaces. The serous membranes which envelop certain organs, as for example the pleura, the pericardium, the peritoneum, supply these membranes with serosity, or serous fluid.

The follicles, a kind of small vesicles placed in the interior of the integuments and mucous membranes, give out a viscid humour, called sebaceous or mucous secretion.

The glands, at once the most important and the most complicated of the secreting organs, furnish peculiar products having no connection with one another. They are formed by a great number of vessels which pass with certain nerves into a cellular or parenchymatous tissue. The product of the secretion issues by an isolated duct, which from its function is called an excretory duct. The liver, the kidneys, the spleen, the salivary glands, &c., are such secreting organs.

Amongst the organic secretions are :—

1. The serum, or serosity, which is separated by serous membranes, which facilitate movement of one surface on another, and prevent the adhesion to other parts of the organs thus invested.

This humour is reabsorbed in proportion to its formation; and the accumulation of it, due to an excess of secretion over absorption, or to a defective correspondence between secretion and absorption, occasions dropsy.

2. Synovial fluid, a humour very similar to the last, intended to make the movements of articulatory surfaces smooth.

3. Fat, the different humours of the eye, &c., belong to this class of secretions.

Excremental Secretions.—The only one necessary to indicate is the urine, secreted by the kidneys, organs shaped like a bean, placed on each side of the vertebral column, and very complicated in structure.

Formed in the kidneys, the urinary fluid is conveyed by the ureters into the bladder, whence it is expelled after a certain quantity is accumulated.

Functional Secretions.—Amongst these are the saliva, secreted by the salivary glands already mentioned; the bile, a greenish-yellow liquid, viscid, bitter, necessary to digestion, secreted by the liver, which is situated in the right hypochondrium, and which is the largest of all the glandular organs.

The tears, elaborated by a special apparatus situated in the internal angle of the eye, and called the lachrymal gland; the pancreatic juice, milk, &c., are also functional secretions.

FUNCTIONS OF RELATION.

SENSATION.

Sensation is the function by which the mind receives the different impressions of external objects. The organs which receive and transmit the impressions of external objects are most sensitive in youth, and become enfeebled in old age. These are called the senses.

There are five senses, viz., sight, hearing, smell, taste, and touch.

The eye, organ of sight, is contained in a cavity which from its form is called the orbit. Of an almost spherical form, the globe of the eye is held firm and movable in the orbit by means of six muscles; any want of concert between these muscles causes strabismus or squinting.

The sclerotic, a white fibrous membrane which forms the principal envelope of the eye, is pierced in its anterior aspect by a circular opening, which is filled up by the transparent cornea by which the light peretrates. The iris, which is a contractile division of various colours, divides the interior of the eye into two chambers which communicate by the opening called the pupil. Behind this is placed the crystalline lens, which fulfils the same functions as the glass lens of an optical instrument, and the opacity of which constitutes the malady known as cataract. On the inner surface of the eye is spread the retina, separated from the sclerotic by the choroid membrane, covered by a black pigment which answers the same purpose in the eye as a black curtain in optical instruments. On the retina, formed by the expansion of the optical nerve, the objects which we see are reflected.

The ear is the organ of hearing. The auditory apparatus is divided into three regions, viz., the external ear, the middle, and the internal; the last two being contained within the skull.

The external ear is composed of the pinna or auricle, which may be considered as an acoustic trumpet; and of the auditory canal, by means of which the sound travels to the other parts of the apparatus.

In the interior, this canal is closed by a very thin membrane called the tympanum. The sound strikes the tympanum and makes it vibrate, transmitting the vibrations to three small bones, and which have been called the malleus or hammer, the incus or anvil, and the stapes or stirrup, and which, in their turn, transmit the sounds to the interior ear in order that the sounds may be transmitted to the expansion of the auditory nerve, which terminates in a pulpy nervous substance without membranous investment. The air reaches the cavity of the tympanum by a canal which opens into the superior lateral surface of the pharynx, and is called the Eustachian tube.

The nose and its dependences are the organs of smell. When the air is drawn in by short and repeated inspirations, the aroma with which it is charged penetrates into the nasal fossæ, lined with a mucous membrane which is called the pituitary membrane. The olfactory nerve is spread on this membrane, and receives the impressions produced by odours.

The tongue is the principal organ of taste, which is perfected by the habit of comparison, and is weakened by the use of too irritating food.

The skin is the seat of touch, which is the more developed in proportion to the fineness of the skin, and as the part which touches is the more capable of moulding itself on the object it touches.

THE VOICE AND SPEECH.

Speech, as we have already said, is one of the great characteristics of man, who alone has the faculty of expressing his thoughts by means of sound. Several animals can make sounds, and consequently have a voice, but in none except man is there to be found an articulate voice, viz., speech. The larynx is the organ which produces vocal sounds, which, modified by the tongue, lips, and palate, is called speech. This organ, situated about the middle of the neck under the skin, and in front of the œsophagus, is continuous below with the trachea. Its external opening is at the lower part of the throat.

The upper opening of the larynx, covered when necessary by the epiglottis, as for example at the instant of deglutition, is about the width of ten lines, and is called the glottis.

The larynx proper is composed of cartilages, cartilaginous fibres, numerous muscles, and a mucous membrane; the cartilage which is the most interesting to study is the thyroid, commonly known as Adam's apple.

The cricoid cartilage is situated above and in front of the preceding; the aritenoid cartilage is behind.

It has been long a matter for discussion whether the larynx should be compared to a wind instrument, or to a string instrument. The question is not yet quite decided, but it is becoming more general to consider it as a key instrument.

The voice, as such, is the effect of the expiration of the air, which produces sound as it passes the glottis. When the vocal sound undergoes modifications, such as those of intonation, intensity, &c., this phenomenon, called the modulated voice or song, is the consequence of the raising or lowering the diameter, &c., of the lips and the glottis.

The articulated voice, that is to say speech, requires other organs; when the vocal sound is produced in the larynx, it is, so to speak, seized and manipulated by the tongue, the lips, the throat, &c., and these subject it to the modifications which distinguish speech from voice, and which enable us to give out our thoughts with so much rapidity.

Stammering is a perversion of pronunciation, the cause of which is almost unknown ; dumbness is the impossibility of speaking, an infirmity mostly due to deafness, which necessarily prevents the formation of sounds of which no idea can be had. This may be complicated by a faulty conformation of the tongue.

Ventriloquism is not, as is generally supposed, the faculty of speaking from the stomach, but simply that of being able to produce a deep and ruffled voice ; it can be acquired by much practice aided by an extensile and flexible larynx, by which voices of different tones and qualities can be imitated.

SLEEP.

If sensation and muscular action are exercised for too long a time, this incessant expenditure of force would not fail sooner or later to injure the individual, and would put a speedy end to his existence. Life could not be sustained on these terms, and nature has provided against such exhaustion by suspending for a certain time the action of our voluntary organs, and thus allowing the human machine to repair its strength. This daily arrest of conscious existence is called sleep.

While sleep lasts, the functions of relation are suspended. Even circulation and respiration are to a slight extent suppressed ; but the functions of assimilation do not by any means cease from their proper action : these work on and continue without interruption their active work of repairing the forces of the organs, and it would seem that the whole organic activity is concentrated into them.

What is the original cause of sleep? Physiology has not been able to tell us ; we only know that fatigue, silence, monotonous sounds, inaction, and weakness provoke sleep.

With children sleep is more prolonged, because young life is characterized by heightened activity and consequently a rapid expenditure of strength. In old age it is light or intermittent. An adult in good health requires six or seven hours' sleep.

It must not be supposed that sleep is always accompanied by perfect repose of the organs, senses, and movements. So far is this from being the case, that we know that even a person who sleeps very quietly will never awake in the same position that he was in when he went to sleep.

Intelligence itself works during sleep ; it associates and combines ideas often in the most foolish way, but sometimes sensibly. It shows us fantastic things, imaginary perils, makes us in turns frightened, hopeful, saddened, or joyful ; and of all these ideas there only remains on awaking a vague remembrance, and often none whatever. We then say we have been dreaming.

Some persons talk in their sleep ; some even rise, dress, and go out of the house, carefully opening and shutting doors, and after doing different things during their walk return to bed, and wake without the slightest remembrance of what they have done. This state is called somnambulism. Marvellous stories are told about this, but they must not be entirely credited.

Somnambulists in their sleep expose themselves to almost as much danger as those who are awakened. Some have been known to throw themselves out of a window under the impression that they were going out of a door. If these persons often avoid those dangers into which persons fall while in their waking state, this results from their passive state not allowing them to perceive the actual danger to which they are exposed, or to judge of its extent. Their slumber thus protects them from the nervous panic which is in itself a frequent cause of accident in the coolest persons.

LOCOMOTION.

Locomotion is the faculty by which all voluntary movement is accomplished, whether it be to escape from danger or to bring us closer to an object which interests us, to grasp it or to take possession of it; shortly, it is the faculty of establishing or avoiding contact with surrounding objects.

The principal agents of locomotion are the bones and muscles; the former are the passive organs, while the second are active, the movement of the bones being entirely dependent on muscular contraction.

Movements.—The movements of which man is capable are of infinite variety. I will not attempt the examination of them all, which would be beyond the limits of my design; I will simply indicate the mechanism of the progressive movements, that is to say, walking, running, jumping, and swimming.

Walking.—In this mode of progression, which is the most ordinary and which can be continued for the greatest length of time, man is standing upright and moves by each leg alternately. The weight of the body is supported by the leg which is resting on the ground, whilst the other is carried forward through the contraction of the muscles and the bending of the joints. When the foot, being carried to a greater or less distance in different persons, is placed on the ground, we bend the body forward so as to be able to lift the leg which is behind, and to perform the same operation as the preceding. Walking is accomplished by a succession of these movements, and is faster in proportion to the rapidity with which the legs are raised and the distance which is left between one foot and another.

Jumping is the movement by which man can project himself certain distances horizontally or vertically and consists in the sudden and rapid extension of the joints after they have been bent. In jumping, it is necessary to imitate the action of an elastic ring which springs suddenly back on being bent. The legs take the largest share in jumping, and it is for this reason that the calves become very much developed in those persons who cultivate this kind of action, as in the case of dancers.

Running belongs to the same description of movement as walking and jumping.

Swimming.—This mode of progression is not natural to man, and he cannot continue it for any length of time. It is an art which may or may not be acquired.

TEMPERAMENT.

The predominance of a certain system of organs on account of a more or less conspicuous difference in moral or physical constitution, forms what is called temperament, of which there are four kinds, viz., sanguine, bilious, nervous, and lymphatic. Nowhere is there found an entirely unmixed specimen of any one of these temperaments ; the definition of which is based on characteristics which are variable in the same person, but can be easily recognized. Consequently, in describing each variety we must suppose those characteristics to be united in an ideal subject which are distributed among different individuals.

Sanguine Temperament.—This results from the predominance of the circulatory system, of which the signs are a quick, frequent, and regular pulse ;

firm, well-developed and rounded muscles; a high fresh colour; medium size.

Psychological Indications.—Great sensitiveness, quick perceptions, good memory, bright, lively disposition, and a tendency to amorous passion.

The athletic temperament—which is an exaggeration of the preceding—is principally distinguished by much greater strength, the muscular system being so much developed that it seems to predominate over the rest.

BILIOUS TEMPERAMENT.—This is caused by the superabundance of bile. The following are its distinguishing features: black hair, yellowish skin, strong, hard, and frequent pulse, muscles firmly developed, and sharp, incisive movements.

Psychological Indications.—Precocious intelligence, irritability, inclination to perseverance, courage, audacity, firmness, often dissimulation.

The melancholic temperament, which is an exaggerated form of biliousness, is distinguished by a dull imagination, and a contradictory disposition.

LYMPHATIC TEMPERAMENT.—Sluggish intelligence, deficient imagination, moderately strong passions, little activity, courage, or perseverance.

NERVOUS TEMPERAMENT.—Physical signs: a pale colour, general emaciation, soft muscles, a thready and frequent pulse.

Psychological Indications.—Lofty ideas, quick sensibility, prompt determination, mobile and imperious disposition, leading to a studious or sedentary life.

The duration of life is not fixed to any special limit. A partial discord between the laws which regulate life causes illness, and greater disorder leads to death, because new laws of matter opposcd to the law of vitality assert themselves. Putrefaction is a sure sign of this last state. It would be absurd to say that life ceases through the destruction of our organism; the cause of death is the cessation of that vital essence called animated existence, that is to say, of the mutual harmony between the sensitive activity of the soul and the activity of matter.

Physiologists who hold a contrary opinion, must find some way of describing those organic lesions which occur in an individual whose life suddenly ceases after some unexpected joy, or a great fright, or electric shock, the effects of a very violent poison, and other analogous causes which can entirely and instantly arrest that power which during the course of existence has been able to resist disease.

RECAPITULATION AND CONCLUSION.

The description of diseases, and the manner in which they should be treated by Electro-Homœopathy, are given in the following table in the same order employed in the register of the Pathogenesis of a Homœopathic medicine. And this order follow the organs of the body—head, eyes, ears, nose, face, &c., to the feet; preceded by general conditions not reparable to any local centre—such as sleep, fever, &c. Several remedies, instead of only one, are indicated in one disease, because it may be that the remedy by means of which the cure must be effected may not be capable of meeting the special peculiarities of every case. In the treatment of all diseases Scrofoloso should be given to all persons with a tendency to the lymphatic temperament; and Angioitico remedies to those of a sanguine temperament: in other words, all treatment must be based upon one of these two specifies. In order to use this materia medica successfully, this fundamental principle must never be overlooked. It will be found useful to consult the following descriptions, which give the treatment suitable to each case.

Besides the special lines of treatment which aro distinctly indicated, and from which variations may be found advisable according to discretion, the treatment must always commence with one of the primary remedies which are referred to in the several sections; passing to the others when experience—which may be gained either in a few minutes or a few days, according to the case—has shown that the primary remedy is insufficient.

When taking different remedies alternately for the same case, they can be taken in different ways; thus one remedy may be taken the first day, another the second, a third on the third day. This method of alternation is preferable in chronic cases. In acute diseases, on the contrary, one remedy should be taken during the first four hours of the morning, another during the next four, and a third afterwards for the same length of time. Another way of alternating—which is usually preferable—consists in taking in rotation one teaspoonful of each of the three remedies in dilution. The effect of the remedies is electric, and instantaneous—so much so, that if a second remedy is taken five minutes after the first, the effect of the first has been already attained, and is not interfered with by that of the second.

This instantaneous effect of remedies can be proved in the cases where pain is present. Suppose, for example, that in a case of spasms of the uterus, if the patient drinks one teaspoonful of a glassful of water in which one globule of Canceroso has been dissolved, the pain will instantly disappear.

When several remedies are being used at the same time, care should be taken that the one most applicable to the disease shall not be left out. If a remedy is used which is not suitable to the disease, it will do no harm, but will produce no effect, in which case another remedy must immediately be substituted, or else the dose changed. During treatment it is by no means necessary to follow any special diet. Good wine makes the remedies more efficacious. Those who care to diet themselves may do so; indeed, it is very important in serous diseases that the patient should be under a milk diet whilst under Electro-Homœopathy.

It should be remembered that the effect of a remedy is equally manifested when applied externally; and when employed both internally and externally the effect is double, and the result is more rapidly obtained.

If a disease yields to the action of a remedy the dose must be increased, because the remedies are similar, *i.e.*, homœopathic. For the same reason, when the disease is grave and violent the dose must be diminished. In desperate cases, however, doses of forty globules at a time may be given.

When curative reaction has once set in treatment should not be interrupted, to avoid the danger of relapse. To prevent any interruption, dry globules may be taken at meal-time.

The treatment should last not only until the disappearance of the symptoms of the disease, but till the disappearance of the cause; hence the necessity of continuing even after apparent cure, a less persistent treatment—as, for example, several globules in wine at meal time, especially after a serious disease.

In desperate cases, instead of the first dilution, forty or fifty globules may be given in a glass, and forty or fifty drops of White or Blue Electricity. Continuous pain, apoplexy, malignant fevers, have been subdued by taking one hundred drops of White or Blue Electricity.

Blue Electricity stops hæmorrhage, and even heals divided arteries.

Electricity applied to the centre of the skull often produces strong effects, because by acting on the brain, the centre of all the nerves, the whole of the organism is acted upon.

Whoever wishes to practise Electro-Homœopathy must firmly grasp these ideas, and follow these general principles.

ABBREVIATIONS.

S. stands for SCROFOLOSO$_1$, or ANTISCROFOLOSO$_1$.
S_2 stands for SCROFOLOSO$_2$, or ANTISCROFOLOSO$_2$.
S_3 stands for SCROFOLOSO$_3$, or ANTISCROFOLOSO$_3$.
S_4 stands for SCROFOLOSO$_4$, or ANTISCROFOLOSO$_4$.
S_5 stands for SCROFOLOSO$_5$, or ANTISCROFOLOSO$_5$.
S_6 stands for SCROFOLOSO$_6$, or ANTISCROFOLOSO$_6$.

C. stands for CANCEROSO$_1$, or ANTICANCEROSO$_1$.
C_2 stands for CANCEROSO$_2$, or ANTICANCEROSO$_2$.
C_3 stands for CANCEROSO$_3$, or ANTICANCEROSO$_3$.
C_4 stands for CANCEROSO$_4$, or ANTICANCEROSO$_4$.
C_5 stands for CANCEROSO$_5$, or ANTICANCEROSO$_5$.
C_{10} stands for CANCEROSO$_{10}$, or ANTICANCEROSO$_{10}$.
T.B. stands for CANCEROSO T.B., or ANTICANCEROSO T.B.

A. stands for ANGIOITICO$_1$, or ANTIANGIOITICO$_1$.
A_2 stands for ANGIOITICO$_2$, or ANTIANGIOITICO$_2$.
A_3 stands for ANGIOITICO$_3$, or ANTIANGIOITICO$_3$.

L. stands for LINFATICO, or ANTILYMPHATIC.

P. stands for PETORALE$_1$, or PECTORAL$_1$.
P_2 stands for PETORALE$_2$, or PECTORAL$_2$.
P_3 stands for PETORALE$_3$, or PECTORAL$_3$.
P_4 stands for PETORALE$_4$, or PECTORAL$_4$.

F. stands for FEBRIFUGO$_1$.
F_2 stands for FEBRIFUGO$_2$.

Ven. stands for Venereo, or Antivenereo.
Ver. stands for $Vermifugo_1$.
Ver_2 stands for $Vermifugo_2$.

R.E. stands for Red Electricity.
Y.E. stands for Yellow Electricity.
W.E. stands for White Electricity.
B.E. stands for Blue or Angioitic Electricity.
G.E. stands for Green Electricity.

For the points for the application of the Electricities see the plate at the end of the book.

Dil.=dilution. alt.=alternately.

DISEASES OF THE BLOOD.

All diseases of the blood are caused—

1. By excess, or rather determination and flow of blood to one part at the expense of other parts; or,

2. By the reverse condition; or, by

3. Impoverishment of the blood.

From excess, or superabundance of blood, proceed all tendencies to active congestion, cerebral, pulmonary, expectoration of blood, congestive hæmorrhage, varicose veins.

Congestion, or stagnation of blood, may be active or passive.

Active, if it is caused by exuberance of vitality; *passive*, if it is caused by relaxation, want of tone, or inertia of the blood-vessels. These are the causes of stagnation in any particular part.

Diseases dependent upon excess of blood should be treated by very small doses, the second or third dilutions.

Treatment.—Dil. A., and very light compresses, often re-dipped, over the heart, made by dissolving 2 globules of A^3 in a tablespoonful of water.

Diseases arising from deficiency of blood, or sluggish circulation, are passive congestions—congestion of the lungs, pneumonia, diseases of the heart, varicose veins. These diseases are cured, or allayed, by ordinary or reduced doses of A.; or of A^2 alt. S. (*See* Apoplexy, Expectoration of Blood, Lung Diseases, &c.)

Anæmia.

Poverty of blood. Anæmic persons are pale, flabby: their flesh is flaccid, of a waxen tint; the gums and lips are scarcely reddened to a rose tint; the pulse is feeble; the least exertion produces oppressed beating and palpitations. In women or young girls, an abundant leucorrhœa often complicates this condition.

Treatment.—Anæmia, as a form of indolent circulation and poverty of blood, is cured in lymphatic constitutions by S. in dilution. The same remedy at meals. Baths of L. alt. A^3. Application of R. E. alt. Y. E. to the solar plexus, pit of stomach, and to the sympathetic, to the stomach, occiput, and great sympathetic centre.

In Angioitics, Dil. A. alt. L. or S. Same remedies in the wine or at meals. Baths of A. Unctions of A^2 to the heart. Application of B. E.

In women with leucorrhœa, Dil. A. alt. C. second dilution. One globule of C^5 every hour. Baths of A^2 alt. C^5. Unctions of F^2 to the hypochondria.

Chlorosis.

A condition dependent upon anæmia, or want of red blood. The most frequent causes are weakness of constitution, lymphatic temperament, want of nourishing food, deficient exercise, too frequent excitement of passion, thwarted affections, amenorrhœa.

Treatment.—Dil. S. alt. A. One globule of C^5 dry, every hour. Application of W. E. to the pit of the stomach, to the sympathetic, the solar plexus, the occiput, and of B. E. to the heart. Baths of A^2. L. C^5. Unctions of F^2 to the hypochondria. In obstinate cases, Dil. C.

Chorea (St. Vitus's Dance).

A kind of convulsive condition, almost continuous (except during sleep), characterized by irregular and involuntary movements, either confined to one set of limbs or to one only, or to special muscles of the face.

Treatment.—Dil. S. alt. C^5 second or third dilution. Application of R. E. alt. Y. E. to the sympathetic, solar plexus, occiput, and dorsal spine. Baths of C^5 (60 to 80 globules to each), or S^5 or W. E. Unctions of C^5 to the whole head, and of A^2 to the heart.

HÆMORRHAGE.

Hæmorrhage is the name given to any flow of blood from the vessels which should contain it, whatever the cause, and whether the fluid escapes externally, or is discharged into the interior of the body, or infiltrates among the tissues. Hæmorrhages are divided into traumatic and spontaneous. The former are the result of wounds produced by some body which divides the vessels; the latter follow upon the influence of organic modifications more or less appreciable. Spontaneous hæmorrhages are so called not because they arise without cause, but because the causes bringing them on are obscure, and sometimes completely hidden. These hæmorrhages have been divided into symptomatic and essential. The former form part of a disorder in which they occur only as one symptom; the latter are not symptoms of any known previous disease, and appear to constitute of themselves the whole morbid state. According to the circumstances under which they appear, they are again divided into active or sthenic, and passive or asthenic. The former occur in strong and plethoric persons, and are preceded by signs of congestion towards the organ which is to be the seat of the flow of blood, and are accompanied by a quasi-febrile action which ceases with the hæmorrhage; the latter, affecting weak and cachectic subjects, have no premonitory symptoms, and are unaccompanied by any reaction.

There are other sub-divisions with which it is equally useful to be acquainted. Thus, when the blood comes to the surface immediately after leaving the vessels, the hæmorrhage is called external. It is called internal when the blood is effused and remains for a longer or shorter period in a cavity in the interstices of the tissues.

When internal hæmorrhage occurs in the interior of certain organs, as the brain, lungs, &c., it is often called apoplexy; under other circumstances it is called an infiltration of blood. It often happens that hæmorrhage occurs at shorter or longer intervals, and sometimes regularly. In this case, it often becomes a necessity of the organism, and its suppression might cause more or less serious disorder. This kind of hæmorrhage is called constitutional.

When hæmorrhage is periodical, it ordinarily occurs in the same organ; if it is effected by other means, which is rare, it is said to be vicarious. When it seems to replace a normal hæmorrhage, as menstruation, or an abnormal hæmorrhage which has become habitual, it is said to be derived or metastatic. Finally, it is called critical when, occurring in the course of acute or chronic disease, it is followed by an advantageous change in the condition of the patient. As to traumatic hæmorrhages, they are either arterial, venous, or capillary, according to the nature of the vessels involved.

Treatment.—A. in dilution, second dilution. Compresses of A3 and B. E.

Varices.

Varicose veins, ulcers, or wounds; varicose state in rheumatism. (*See* also Phlebitis.)

Treatment.—A. Dil. or A3 alt. C. second dilution. The same remedies at meals, 5 or 10 globules alternately. Compresses of A3, or of C5. Application of B. E. on the varicose parts.

When varicose condition is consequent upon congestion of the liver, A. alt. F. should be given.

Many cases of varicose veins are cured in two months by A. and A^2, internally and applied as compresses.

Phlebitis.

Inflammation of the venous system, forming hard and painful cords.

Treatment.—A. in dilution, or A. alt. S. first dilutions. The same remedies alt. dry, twice a day in a dose of 5 globules. Compresses of A^3 or B. E. on the diseased veins. Unctions of A^3 to the heart. Baths of A. or A. alt. L.

Morbid Obesity.

Disordered nutrition of the adipose tissues, producing an accumulation of fat in all parts of the body, and especially under the skin. It is principally over the abdomen, over the upper part of the back, on the hips and on the mammary glands, that obesity is developed.

The exaggerated development of adipose tissue, giving enormous volume to the body, extends to the interior of of the body, around the larynx, the lungs, the intestines, the liver, and hinders the free action of all the functions. Obesity is a serious predisposing cause of saccharine diabetes. The causes are a lymphatic temperament, self-indulgence, sedentary habits, excessive rest in bed, good living, abuse of fatty food, decline of life in either sex.

Treatment.—Abstinence from the predisposing causes. Dil. A. alt. L. or Ven. alt. A^3. 20 globules dry of A^3. Baths of C^5. alt. A^3. Application of R. E. alt. Y. E. to the occiput, the sympathetic, and the solar plexus. Unctions of F^2 to the hypochondria. Baths of L.

Marasmus.

Wasting away, excessive emaciation, loss of fat, muscular fibre, and tissue generally; loss of appetite, accompanied by dry cough which comes on later, and indicates the approach of phthisis.

Treatment.—S. in dilution alt. C. second dilution. Application of R. E. alt. Y. E. to the solar plexus and grand sympathetic. W. E. over the head.

Rickets.

Softening and distortion of the bones, arising from a serious degeneration in the lymph.

Treatment.—Dil. C. S. $A._3$ first dilution. The same remedies at meals (4 globules, alternately). Baths of L. or Ven. Unctions of C^5 to the back and the head. Application of R. alt. Y. E. to the great sympathetic, the solar plexus, the occiput, and the pit of the stomach.

Atrophy.

Wasting, general or partial, of a limb or an organ, or of its essential constituents, muscles, blood-vessels, bones. Marasmus is atrophy of the cellular and muscular tissues.

Treatment.—Dil. S. Application of R. E. or R. E. alt. Y. E. to the nerves related to the atrophied parts, and to the great sympathetic. In obstinate cases C. or A^2. Baths of C^5. Unctions of F^2 to the hypochondria. Baths of W. E. Two tablespoonfuls to each bath. Compresses of W. E.

Scrofula.

A disease characterized by lesion both of the bones and the soft tissues, but especially by enlargement of the lymphatic glands under the lower jaw and down the neck, the groins, the axillæ, &c.

The chief scrofulous diseases are those of the glands, diseases and eruptions of the skin, cold or indolent tumours, abscesses, ulcers and fistulæ. Most cases of ophthalmia, many diseases causing alteration in the bones and cartilages, tuberculization, are of scrofulous nature. S. supplemented if necessary by C¹ and C5 cover all these diseases. For treatment, see the separate diseases.

Scurvy.

A disease characterized chiefly by general feebleness, hæmorrhages in different parts, livid patches of ecchymosis or blood-stains, swelling and easy bleeding of the gums.

The prolonged action of cold appears to be one of the most effective causes of scurvy. This disease also appears especially in vessels at sea, if they are deprived of fresh meat and fresh vegetables.

Depressing emotion, want of cleanliness, the exclusive use of salted food, excessive fatigue, or unusual and unaccustomed inactivity, are contributory causes in the development of this disease.

Aversion to every kind of movement is one of the first symptoms of scurvy. To this we may add, languor, heaviness and pains in the limbs, less frequently general swelling with hard tumours in the muscles of the calf and of the thigh, with drawing up of the legs; the action of the heart and the pulsation of the arteries are slow and feeble. The patient faints at the least movement; at all points, blood may escape from the enclosing vessels, and became infiltrated beneath the cuticle or skin, producing subcutaneous hæmorrhage, or hæmorrhage under the mucous membranes, or breaking out of bleeding in old scars, or in cicatrized wounds and ulcers in the skin. To the ordinary symptoms of scurvy we may also refer the livid swelling of and the bloody oozing from the gums; œdema of the limbs; pallor, lividity and puffy condition of the face, lowered tone of the moral and physical faculties; difficult digestion; colic; oppressed respiration, loss of heat, offensiveness or fœtor of the breath.

Amidst these serious troubles the intellectual faculties

are usually intact; but there is great moral depression, despair, nostalgia or pining, and sometimes tendency to suicide. After a varied duration, scurvy terminates either by a cure or by death. Death results either from a paroxysm of oppressed breathing and suffocation, or in a fainting fit; or else patients gradually fade away and sink from exhaustion.

Treatment.—The treatment of scurvy is above all things hygienic. For instance, a dry air, warm clothing, good animal and vegetable food, are essential both as preventives and for curative treatment.

C^5 Dil. alt. A^3. Baths of L. Gargles of B. E. **Unctions over the heart and aorta, of A^3, and of F^2 to the hypochondria. Compresses of S^5 and of C^5 over the open bleeding surfaces.**

Adenitis.

Acute or chronic inflammation of lymphatic ganglions or glands. These are the little rounded masses situated in the line of nerves and lymphatic vessels; especially apt to occur in the neck, the groin, the arm-pits, &c.

In *Acute Adenitis* the patient suffers from pain and heat, the skin is inflamed, suppuration is established.

Dil. S. alt. S^5 and L. or A. alt. C.; same remedies at meals. Some spoonfuls of F^1. Baths of C^5 alt. A. or of C^5 alt. A^3. Compresses and unctions of C^5 on the glands. Application of R. E. and Y. E. alternately to the affected nerves.

Chronic Adenitis. The swollen glands are indolent, inactive. If any opening occurs the pus is of thin consistence; and if the cold abscess or ulceration closes it is liable to reopen very soon. As a rule the swelling is in the glands of the neck and jaws.

Treatment.—Dil. S. alt. A. or A. alt. C.; 5 globules of L. in the wine at meals. Baths of L. A^3 C^5. Compresses and unctions of C^5. Compresses of G. E.

SCROFULOUS GLANDS IN THE NECK.

Treatment.—S. or L. in dilution. If they are obstinate, C. in dilution, second dilution. Application of R. E. to the related nerves. Baths of L. C^5. Unctions and compresses of C^5.

SALIVARY GLANDS UNDER THE EARS.

C. in second dilution or A. Compresses and gargles of C^5. Application of R. E. alt. Y. E. on the related nerves. C^5 in dil. alt. A.

DISEASED GLANDS IN THE ABDOMEN: MESENTERIC DISEASE.

(*See* Marasmus.)

Treatment.—Always C., and as before in very small doses.

GENERAL DEBILITY.

A state in which the forces are diminished; it must not be confounded with simple weakness which may be natural to an individual, in contradistinction to the debility which always indicates some profound functional alteration. Weakness is one thing, General Debility another.

Treatment.—Sometimes the mere application of R. E. to the pit of the stomach and to the solar plexus will restore nervous power. If weakness persists we must give, according to the constitution, A. or S. in the first dilution. The same, dry, at meals. Application of R. E. alt. Y. E. to the skull, to the occiput, the sympathetic, the solar plexus, and to the back along the course of the dorsal spine. Baths of S^5 C^5 A^3.

CEREBRAL WEAKNESS.

Through abuse of quinine.

Treatment.—S. in dilution (first glass). Application of R. E. alt. Y. E. to the grand sympathetic, pit of the stomach, occiput, solar plexus, and all the nerves of the head. Baths of C^5 alt. S^2 and of W. E.

Fainting.

Treatment.—10 globules, dry of S. Application of R. E. to the pit of the stomach, to the sympathetic, the occiput, the solar plexus.

Congestions of all Kinds (*of Glands and Tissues*).

Treatment.—S. in dilution alt. A^2 second dilution. The same remedies at meal-time. If necessary C. second dilution. Baths of C^5 A^2 or W. E. Applications of B. E. or R. E. alt. Y. E. to the related nerves. Compresses of A^2 over the heart.

Acute or Chronic Inflammations.

Treatment.—S. internally or externally, and in the case of sanguine temperament A. alt. S. But if there is fever F^1 must of course be used. either alone, or alt. with S. or A. When an inflammatory fever is very violent, begin by treating the fever by itself, give F^1 in spoonfuls, smaller and more frequent according to the violence of the fever, and add F^2 in compresses or unctions to the hypochondria.

The fever subdued, continue F^2 in unction; give S., and if the patient is sanguine, A. alt. S.

Fevers.

We must now refer to a group of diseases which are very important, and which often cause great ravages in the system. These affections, which are usually very grave, have their seat or centre in the stomach, or the intestines, or the liver, without however giving any certain indication that they depend upon any inflammatory condition of these organs. We need hardly say that we allude to various forms of gastric fever, mucous fever, putrid or malignant fever, abdominal typhoid, with or without ulceration of the enteric glands, and with or without rash on the surface.

These diseases, which attack so many victims, are divided into three distinct stages, namely: 1. The inflammatory or invasion stage. 2. The abdominal stage, properly so called, or the gastro-intestinal stage; the tongue being covered with a coating of a yellow, white, or livid colour. 3. The adynamic stage, or exhaustion throughout the entire organism, especially in the functions of the intestines. This is the stage of humoral or fluid decomposition; indicated by the black colour of the tongue, teeth, and lips; by fœtid perspiration, by epistaxis or bleeding from the nose, by intestinal and urinary hæmorrhage, by petechiæ or blood blotches on the skin, which are nothing more than hæmorrhages of the cutaneous capillary vessels. The pulse is always very weak and sometimes insensible. This last phase of intestinal fever only reaches its extreme height in abdominal typhus; while, on the other hand, in bilious and mucous fevers the symptoms are always less alarming, although it is evident that these intestinal disorders have sufficient energy to produce profound disturbance in the organism.

During the first and second stages we must use S. alt. F., or F. alt. A. in the second or third dilution, with unctions of F^2 to the hypochondria, and application of R. E. and Y. E. to the solar plexus, the grand sympathetic, and the pit of the stomach. But in the third stage we must necessarily resort to C^1, 1 globule every hour, and C^5 in unctions and compresses over the abdomen; with application of W. E. or R. E. to the occiput, the grand sympathetic, the solar plexus, along the whole length of the dorsal spine, and on the soles of the feet—this in order to secure the general action of the specific over the whole body. During the course of these diseases complications may arise; among others, cerebral congestion, leading to delirium; disturbance of the spinal cord, with alterations in its motor or sensory functions. But the most frequent complication—arising from the great sympathy which exists between the skin and the gastro-enteric mucous membrane—is miliary eruption, preceded by abundant perspiration; and petechiæ. These are part of the nosology of these diseases. But we need not be too easily discouraged. As soon as we use internally F. alt. S., or S., an immediate amelioration is produced. The great secret of natural law, and the unequivocal proof that treatment is natural, is to produce great results by the use of simple means.

It often happens, especially when we have nervous persons under treatment, of an impressionable and changeable type, that we have to deal with certain gastric disorders, attendant upon adynamic fever. The special characteristic of this singular disease is a remarkably fluctuating state; so that a person who seems at one time to have an excellent appetite and good digestion, loses his appetite all at once, the mouth becomes pasty, the tongue covered with a coating of whitish mucous matter, and clammy features are contracted; everything about the patient indicates a sudden loss of vital force in the functions of the digestive apparatus, and especially in the stomach.

This disorder, which has always resisted various methods of treatment, can be victoriously encountered by F. alt. C., first or second dilution, and unctions of F^2 to the hypochondria, application of W. E. to the sympathetic and solar plexus. We should add also three drops of the same electricity on a lump of sugar, and baths of C5.

Before concluding this short study, which is as practical as it is interesting, we may be permitted to allude to a disorder which is very frequent in children, especially those of lymphatic temperament—we refer to helminthiasis or affections arising from the presence of worms. This is a secondary condition connected with a special irritation of the gastro-enteric mucous membrane, which secretes mucous material capable of nourishing these parasites. This is a cause, in children, of disorders so strange in character, and often so alarming, that it suggests matters for reflection to parents, and often for physicians, if they are not cognizant of the direct cause of these evils. These may be convulsions; spinal irritation, and even epileptic attacks; catalepsy arising from pain seated in the region of the vertebral column, which can only be explained by the direct relations existing between this part of the organism and the nerves of the stomach, which, irritated by the worms, exert a strong influence on the whole nervous system. These disorders of the digestive apparatus of infants cause the pupils to dilate, a blue circle surrounds the eyes, the nose itches, and the general surface is covered with that characteristic pallor which, more than any other symptom, indicates worm disorders. The use of Ver. will dissipate at once the causes and the effects of these curious maladies. This remedy should be taken in the first or second dilution. Dry globules of the same, on the tongue, should be taken at bedtime; baths, unctions, and enemata, especially if epileptic convulsions arise; and unctions of F[2] and C5 to the hypochondria.

Similar treatment is equally efficacious in adults; for it is not only children who have worms—this torment may visit all ages. If there is one resident which more than another is annoying, and causes great injury to the intestines and to the whole nervous system, it is the tænia, or tape-worm. The use of Ver. removes this and all other descriptions of worms. Worms once dead, form a sort of mass which remains fixed in the large intestine. By the use of enemata of the same remedy they may be expelled, and thus the putrid adynamic disorders may be prevented which destroy so many children.

The dose of Ver. may vary from 30 to 40 globules for some days, and as Yellow or Negative Electricity is also a vermifuge, it is well to take 5 or even 10 drops in a teaspoonful of water twice a day.

Often the presence of worms in the intestinal canal neutralizes the action of remedies. Accordingly, if a remedy is ineffectual in a case where it is specifically indicated, we must alternate the use of it with Ver.

CONTINUOUS FEVERS.

In these fevers, the febrile condition lasts during the whole continuance of the fever. They comprise ephemeral fever, inflammatory fever, typhoid fever.

Ephemeral fever, or a fever of short duration, begins with shivering, followed by heat, headache, pains in the loins, lumbago, hot but soft skin, red face, no appetite, much thirst, white tongue, scanty and red urine, constipation, full and frequent pulse.

Treatment.—All fevers are treated with F. internally, and F^2 to the hypochondria in compresses and unctions.

Electricities can be also applied to the occiput, alternating the R. E. and Y. E., or only using the W. E.

Inflammatory fever is similar to the last, but is preceded by giddiness, headaches, bewilderment, and sleepiness.

F. in dilution, second or third dilution, one teaspoonful every 5 minutes. Unctions of F^2 to the hypochondria. In stopping inflammatory fevers at once, the disorder is often, as it were, stamped out, and if some sense of illness is still left, a complete cure is obtained by giving S. or A^3 (second dilution), and unctions of F^2 to the hypochondria.

Typhoid fever is often accompanied by cerebral nervous disorders, and becomes virtually nervous fever.

First period: Fever, intense headache, changed features, stupefied expression, delirium, giddiness, tinnitus or drum-like noise in the ears, bleeding from the nose, a bitter, slimy or insipid taste in the mouth, white tongue, nausea, vomiting, loss of appetite, the abdomen tender and distended, diarrhœa, or constipation.

Second period: The headache diminishes but the stupor increases, the features become fixed, the tongue is covered with a brown coating, which stains the teeth and lips, the abdomen is swollen, the evacuations black, fetid, and involuntary, the urine scanty and brown.

Treatment.—F. in dilution, third dilution; one teaspoonful every 5 minutes. Unctions and compresses of F^2 to the hypochondria, or F. alt. C^5 in unctions and compresses.

Mucous Fever.

The same treatment, second dilution.

Nervous Fever.

The same treatment, second dilution.

Bilious Fever.

The same treatment, second dilution.

Catarrhal Fever.

F. first dilution alt. P^3 second dilution.

Puerperal Fever.

F. second dilution alt. C. second dilution.

Eruptive Fevers.

Variola or small-pox, measles, erysipelas, scarlatina, miliary fever, and nettle-rash. All suppressed eruptions are restored and cured by S. (alone). The more violent and rapid the disorder the more must the dilution be weakened, and the dose repeated, that is teaspoonful doses every few minutes.

Intermittent Fever.

Returning periodically, divided into periods of cold, heat, and perspiration.

Intermittent fevers have been divided into simple, pernicious, irregular, and symptomatic.

An intermittent fever is simple when it is confined to pure and simple feverish attacks. It is pernicious according to the intensity of the cold or perspiration. It is irregular when the attacks are incomplete, or when one or other of the stages, cold, heat, or perspiration, is wanting.

Symptomatic intermittent fevers depend upon some local change.

Treatment.—F. in dilution, first dilution; 20 to 30 tablespoonfuls during the day, while there is no fever, and continued afterwards. A. alt. with F. is sometimes added, and dissipates intermittent fever, especially during the growing age in girls. Also, when fever is the result of some disordered circulation of the blood, A. must be added. A., by restoring the blood to its normal state, counteracts the fever.

Intermittent fevers sometimes leave chronic affections of the liver, which can only be cured by using F. (*see* Febrifugo, page 34).

Scarlatina.

Is an eruptive and contagious fever recognizable by little red points regularly dispersed over the skin, something like mottled shagreen, covering nearly the entire surface of the body and the interior of the mouth. There is also shivering, fever, sore-throat, headache, nausea, sometimes also bleeding at the nose. Scarlatina is distinguished from measles by the invariably accompanying sore throat: moreover, when the scarlatina rash appears in the form of large red patches, like the stains of strawberry juice, no mistake is possible.

Treatment.—All rashes and eruptions, if thrown in (repercussion of rash), are brought back and cured by the use of S.

The more violent the attack, the more must the doses be reduced, and the more frequently repeated—in teaspoonful doses every five minutes S. dil. alt. F. second or third dilution.

If the disease is obstinate, and if the existence of tubercles in the lungs is suspected, or if there is discharge from the ears, or suppuration of the glands of the neck, add C.

The best plan is to stamp out the fever at the outset, by giving F. in teaspoonful doses every ten minutes—even every five minutes if the case is a bad one, using the first, second, or third glass according to the severity of the attack; adding compresses of F^2, often renewed, 10 or 15 globules to the glass. Sometimes we may add an application of R. E. alt. Y. E. to the occiput and the sympathetic; and if the patient has a sanguine temperament we should use B. E.

The same treatment applies to measles and to all specific fevers.

VARIOLA (*see* Fevers).

Fever, lassitude, pains in the kidneys and hips, headache, nausea, vomiting, irritation of the mucous surfaces, delirium. On the third day an eruption of pustules begins; at first hard, then filled with a fluid which is at first transparent, then becomes turbid and purulent; after these have dried up, a depression more or less deep and durable remains.

Treatment.—If there are syphilitic conditions, add Ven. internally and externally in very feeble doses. The *Blear-eyed* state is ordinarily syphilitic, and requires A. internally and externally, alt. Ven. S. alt. Ven. with compresses of A^2, W. E. or B. E.

If there is hæmorrhage in the eye, A. dil. or A^3. Unctions over the whole head of A^3 and C^5. Baths of C^5. Apply B. E. to the occiput, the sympathetic and all the nerve points of the head.

EPIDEMICS.

In case of epidemics, fevers, eruptions, cholera, the regular and daily use of S. cannot be too highly recommended, either diluted or dry, one globule every hour.

Rheumatism.

See the section on Pain. Rheumatism is an excessively vagrant malady, moving from one part to another, seated in muscular and fibrous tissues. It arises from a vice of blood, and it is often replaced by some skin eruption, and returns when the eruption disappears.

Treatment.—If it is accidental it will yield to R. E.; sometimes to R. E. alt. Y. E. and to G. E., if there is pain in the joints. If it returns, it can only be effectually dealt with by internal means. Dil. S. second dilution, 10 globules in wine at meals. Baths of S. or of C5 or A2, or W. E. Compresses of G. E. on the joints and the painful parts.

It is to be observed that in rheumatism S. should be taken in the second dilution if there is no crisis; in the third if there is crisis.

In inveterate cases of rheumatic gout, with nodes, swelling and distortion of the joints, C. internally and C5 externally are very efficacious.

Hysteria: Hysteric Laughing.

Treatment.—Dil. S. second dilution. Application of R. E. alt. Y. E. to the great sympathetic, the solar plexus, and the occiput. Baths of C5.

Arthritis.

Inflammation of the fibrous and serous tissues of the joints: distinguished from gout, because it only attacks one or two joints at the same time.

Treatment.—Dil S. 20 globules of L. dry, on waking. Baths of C5. Compresses of A3 to the heart, and of F2 to the hypochondria. In obstinate cases Dil. C. Application of G. E. to the suffering parts.

ARTICULAR RHEUMATISM.

Pains more or less excruciating in the joints, very generally producing swelling and redness of the affected parts, with more or less high fever. This disease may be complicated by two serious diseases: inflammation of the membrane which surrounds the heart, or of that which forms a coating to the cavities of the heart—pericarditis, and endocarditis.

Treatment.—Dil. A. alt. C. Same remedies at meals. Baths of C^5 and of G. E. Unctions over the heart of A^2, and of F^2 over the hypochondria. 10 globules of Vermifugo before sleep.

The articulations may be the seat of rheumatic gout, of gouty deposit, of general arthritis, of anchylosis, or of caries. In infants, swelling of the joints is generally a sign of rickets. The elbow and knee joints may be the seat of white swelling.

Treatment.—Dil. S. Application of R. E. to the solar plexus, the occiput, the pit of the stomach and the sympathetic. In obstinate cases, C. alt. A. Baths of C^5 or S.

GOUT.

A disease characterized by pain, swelling, and redness of the small joints, nearly always attacking the great toe in the first instance; movable in subsequent attacks, it may spread to the large joints, and cause disorder in most functions of the body, and especially the digestive system.

Treatment.—S. in dilution, first dilution. Application of R. E. to the occiput, sympathetic, and solar plexus. If the joints have been knotty for a long time, C. or C^5 must be given. Baths of C^5 and R. E. Compresses on the cranium and all the painful parts of R. E., W. E., or B. E. Alt. later on with 10 globules dry of C^5 daily; later, 10 globules A^3 and S.; C. alt. A^3 in wine at meal-time (5 to 10 globules).

Several cases of gout have been cured by A. or by A. alt. S. Obstinate gout is often of syphilitic origin, when Ven. in dilution must be added, also in compresses and baths.

ANCHYLOSIS.

Inflammation of the joints, or gout. Is seen also in the fingers. This disease is acute or chronic; it is often the result of a psoric disorder of the skin, and often also it is connected with syphilitic disease.

Treatment.—Must be long continued. Dil. S. or S^2, L., S^5, or C^5. alt. A. (second dilution). One globule of C^5 every hour. Baths of L., C^5, S^5 or W. E. Unctions of F^2 to the hypochondria. Compresses on the articulations of G. E. or B. E. Application of R. E. alt. Y. E. to the solar plexus, pit of the stomach, sympathetic at the stomach, occiput, great sympathetic, and to all the suffering nerves. If the disease is obstinate, C. C^3.

DROPSY.

Infiltration of serous fluid beneath the skin.

Symptoms.—The skin is pallid, swollen, painless; weakness, intense thirst; later, diarrhœa; hardly any urinary secretion. Dropsy may occur after a chill, or any fever, from disease of the heart, and altered state in the urinary secretion. Dropsy (excepting when in the lungs) must be treated with the remedy adapted to the organ attacked by the flow of serous fluid, and in small doses. Tapping or puncture does not cure, it only delays death—sometimes even hastens it when the lower limbs, much swollen, are threatened with gangrene.

Treatment.—The external use of C^5 is indispensable. If the dropsy comes from the liver, use F^1 perseveringly; if from the bronchi, P^1; if from the ovaries, C^1. The action of S^1 may be useful in alternation with these three remedies.

Anasarca, or Œdema.

Infiltration of the cellular tissues with serous fluid—it is properly called general dropsy of this tissue. Patients thus affected have pallor of the skin, and an indolent kind of swelling which gives under the fingers, "pits under pressure," and retains for a certain time the impression thus produced, as if in a wax model: this is especially on the limbs. Besides this there is debility, thirst, and, at a more advanced period, diarrhœa; moreover the urinary secretion is almost absent. This may arise from a chill, or it may follow fever or acute diseases, or arise from a generally cachectic or depraved condition of health.

Treatment.—Dil. S. alt. A., generally in the second dilution. Sometimes F. or C. in the second dilution. Unctions of F^2 to the hypochondria. Friction on the swollen parts with W. E. alt. B. E. Baths of A^2, C^5, L.

In swelling of the hypochondria, take F^1 second dilution. Unctions of F^2 to the swelling. Baths of C^5. Compresses of W. E. on the hypochondria.

Dropsy in the Chest.

Symptoms.—Hardly any pain, oppression, difficult respiration, small and rapid pulse; livid face, swelling of the legs and feet, abnormal bruit or murmur in the heart on auscultation; fluctuation on moving the body.

Treatment.—S. in dilution (weak doses). If the heart is suffering, or the circulation is impeded, A^2 or A^2 alt. S.

If the bronchi are diseased, P^1 or A. alt. P. alt. S. second dilution. If the dropsy is consequent upon disease of the lungs, S^1 alt. C^1 alt. P^1.

Dropsy in the Stomach.

Accumulation of serous fluid in the peritoneal cavity, with uniform swelling.

Treatment.—C^1 in dilution alt. F^1 second dilution. If the heart and blood are affected, A^2 or S alt. A^2 second dilution; if the liver is affected, F^1 alt. S^1 second dilution; if the dropsy originates in the mesenteric glands, C. alt. S. second dilution.

Dropsy of the Ovary.

An affection of slow progress, without pain or much discomfort; the abdomen is swollen on one side only. Later the patient feels a weight in the stomach and in the renal region; constant necessity to urinate or difficulty in so doing; constipation; later, swelling of the lower limbs; short respiration; sometimes extreme oppression. This disease, which is only to be thoroughly recognized by external and internal examination, may continue for many years.

Treatment.—C^5 in dilution alt. F^1 second or third dilution. R. E. on the stomach. Compresses of C^5 on the ovaries.

Hydarthrosis.

Articular dropsy. A disease occasioned by the accumulation of a large quantity of synovial fluid in the capsule of a joint.

Hydarthrosis occurs particularly in the most movable joints, as the knee, foot, wrist, elbow. The most ordinary causes are:—Living in cold and damp places, gouty and rheumatic conditions, wounds in the joints, sprains, violent or extreme exercise, articular concretions, syphilitic virus. The signs are swelling of the joint, with fluctuation; difficulty and even impossibility of movement. When the disorder appears in the knee, the outline of the kneecap disappears because of the swelling and the distension of the synovial membrane, which surrounds the bones on all sides.

Treatment.—S. in dilution or A. alt. C^1. Baths of C^5.

Unctions on the affected parts of C4. If the cause is a syphilitic virus, add Ven. internally and externally.

Poisoning.

If the poisoning is accidental, or owing to some allopathic medicine, such as iodine, mercury, &c., the first dilution of S. or dry globules are used: 20 if the poison is acting rapidly. If slowly, and if there has been time for the blood to be affected, the same remedy will answer (20 globules dry), then the first dilution of C., and one globule of C5 every hour. In case of poisonous fungi or other venomous articles of food, if vomiting has not occurred spontaneously, the patient must be made to vomit, even before taking a remedy, by the use of tepid water medicated with S.

One glassful of the first dilution of S. is generally necessary for all poisonings and their consequences; one globule of C5 every hour. Baths of S2 alt. A2 alt. C5. Application of W. E. to the pit of the stomach, the solar plexus, the occiput, and the gastric sympathetic.

Antidotes.—If a wrong remedy has been taken, it is antidoted by the same remedy in the second or third dilution. In general, we descend one or two degrees below the dose which has caused aggravation. Against the over-use of a remedy, vinegar or lemon-juice.

Carbuncle: Malignant Pustule.

A nodulated excrescence, a tumour very hard and painful, not much raised, with a deep red margin, and livid vesicles in the centre, which develop into a slough black as charcoal. It is a disease which may arise from contact with animals suffering from carbuncular or similar disease.

Treatment.—Dil. S. alt. S.; same remedies dry, 5 globules at each meal. One globule of C5 every hour. Daily baths of C5 alt. S. or A2. Unctions or compresses of C5 alt.

A^2 alt. S. Application of R. E. alt. Y. E. to the related nerves.

SIMPLE OR NON-MALIGNANT ANTHRAX.

Inflammation resembling that of a boil in several parts of the cellular tissue. A simple boil only affects one part at a time of this tissue.

At the outset there is swelling, pains at the seat of disease; soon the tumour increases, becomes very hard, painful, throbbing, and of a deep red colour. There is fever, shivering, loss of appetite, diarrhœa or constipation, nausea, and sometimes vomiting.

Treatment.—Subdue the fever by F^1 in dilution and unctions of F^2 to the hypochondria. Same treatment as the prior case.

ABSCESS.

Under this name we include abscess as ordinarily understood, whitlow, boils, carbuncles, styes, and in general all collections of pus in an abnormal or artificial cavity.

At the commencement of abscess, the patient suffers from rigors or shivering attacks, fever, agitation; the pus is thick and creamy, of a greenish yellow colour. Abscesses may arise in any part of the body, and be either deep or superficial.

Cold abscess never occurs except in lymphatic subjects. It develops slowly, is not preceded by any inflammatory process, and the pus is formed without any precedent pain. As a rule, the pus in these abscesses is very liquid.

Treatment.—In lymphatic cases, S. dil. alt. C. dil. Globules of the same taken in wine at meals; baths of C^5 alternately with S^5. Unctions and compresses of C^5 on the affected parts. Application of R. E. alternately with Y. E. on the contiguous nerves, and to the sympathetic.

In Sanguine or Angioitic cases, S. dil. alt. C. dil.; and in obstinate cases, A. alt. C. Baths of A^3 alternately with

C^5. Unction and compresses of the same remedies; application of B. E.

Inflammatory or acute abscesses are always attended with tumefaction, redness, lancinations, and heat, fever with shivering. The pus is thick, heavy, and greenish yellow in colour.

Dil. A. alt. Dil. C. The same remedies at meal-times; one globule of C^5 every hour. Baths alternately of A^3 and C^5. Unctions and compresses of A^3 alternately with C^5. Unctions over the heart of A^3. Unctions to the hypochondria of F^2. Application of R. E. alternately with Y. E. to the solar plexus, pit of the stomach, to the sympathetic at the stomach, the occiput, and the cervical sympathetic centre. On the skull 5 drops of B. E. Subdue the fever also with some spoonfuls of F^2 second dilution.

Congestive abscess results from gangrene or caries of the bones. It forms a fistulous canal, which, starting from the seat of disease, carries along the abnormal secretion which results from the caries. The pus is serous, semi-fluid, and often becomes putrid in contact with the air.

Dil. C^1 second dilution; the same remedy at meals; one globule of C^5 every hour; baths of C^5. Applications alternately of R. E. and Y. E. to the solar plexus, pit of the stomach, the occiput, and great sympathetic. Unction of F^2 to the hypochondria. Compresses of C^4.

Boils: Furuncles.

A light inflammation seated in the cellular tissue. This condition terminates either by resolution or suppuration.

Treatment.—Dil. S. alt. A. Same remedies at meals. Baths of C^5 alt. A^2 alt. S^5 or L. Compresses of C^5. Application of R. E. alt. Y. E. to the occiput, sympathetic, and to the related nerves.

Boils under the orbit require Dil. A. alt. S. Compresses of C^5 alt. A^2. Application of R. E. alt. Y. E. above and below the orbit.

Gangrene.

Or death of an isolated part of the organism, called dry, or moist—dry, when the parts affected are dry and hard; and moist, if they are soft, as if putrified, and break up at the slightest pressure. Around the gangrenous part an inflammatory process is going on, the living part trying to detach itself from and throw off the dead. If this proves successful, a suppurating wound is left, leaving a scar; if unsuccessful, the grangene encroaches upon the living part, and soon causes death.

Treatment.—C. in dilution, second dilution. 20 globules of C5 on waking. Baths of S5 and C5. Unctions and compressions of C5. Compresses of W. E. or G. E. Application of R. E. alt. Y. E. on the related nerves. Pomade of C5 crushed and mixed with fresh butter is excellent for deep ulcerating bedsores and gangrenous destruction on the sacrum. This also is applicable to all external gangrenes.

Ulcers: of all Kinds.

Treatment.—S1 and C., or C. and C5 internally and externally. Apply G. E. (*See* Cancer, Scirrhus, Skin, Venereal Diseases.)

Vaccination.

For poisoning consequent upon the use of impure vaccine lymph.

Treatment.—S. internally, and baths of L.

Fistulas of Scrofulous or Psoric origin.

S. in dilution. Applications of R. E. on the nerves related to the disorder; in obstinate cases, S. alt. C. Baths of C5 or L. Applications of R. E. alt. Y. E. to the related nerves.

Lachrymal Fistula.

Ulceration in the canal at the internal angle of the eye.

Treatment.—S. or C. Applications of R. E. to the occiput, sympathetic nerve, sub and supra orbital regions.

Fistula of the Gums.

Treatment.—S. in dilution or C. Gargles of L. or C5, or W. E. Application of R. E. to the related nerves.

CANCEROUS AND GLANDULAR OR OTHER TUMOURS.

Cancer.

A substance of unknown origin, with a tendency tc spread continually and destroy surrounding parts. If it is removed by operation, it almost always returns, either in the same place or elsewhere. Cancer is distinguished from many other tumours, and among the rest from Cancroid tumours (corroding ulcers), by the existence of a peculiar cell in its tissues, only to be recognized by the microscope. And while in other tumours cachexia—breaking up or degeneration of the constitution—is not constant, in cancer it is invariable, and arises from absorption into the blood of the cancerous veins, and a generally poisoned condition of the constitution. The ordinary lancinating pains may be absent; usually they do not present themselves at the outset, or in the stage of deposition. They begin to appear with the stage of extension, and increase in severity to the last.

Principal Types of Cancer.

1. *Encephaloid Cancer.* A soft variety, with a substance resembling brains or marrow; the most frequent of all forms.

2. *Gelatinous or Colloid Cancer.* Softer even than the preceding. In this case a kind of transparent jelly, colour-

less or yellowish, sometimes rather red, something like glue or gelatine, is infiltrated into the cancerous tissues.

3. *Hematoid Cancer.* In this cancer the diseased mass has a hæmorrhagic character, and bleeding is frequent.

4. *Melanic Cancer* (black cancer). In this type a black colouring matter is added to the cancerous tissue, and gives it a tint varying from grey to black.

5. *Scirrhus Cancer, or simply Scirrhus.* Hard cancer; the hardness varying from that of cartilage to that of stone—stony cancer. Whether the cancer is more or less hard, or more or less soft, does not alter its essential character. The blood disease is the same, and is determined by the existence of the cancer cell.

Ulceration does not always exist even in cancers of the breast and of the stomach. In cancer of the skin it is often absent. In cancers of the bones and of the eye it comes later, and is due only to the development of the tumour. It is very rare in cancer of the liver, the testicles, the ovaries, or the kidneys, and softening in more than half the cases does not occur.

Often the cancerous disease manifests itself by the appearance, either around the principal cancer, or in other places, of a quantity, more or less, of secondary tumours. But in some cases this effect does not show itself, and yet the cancerous disease is not less active in extending itself through the whole mass of the blood, and death results more from blood-poisoning and blood-decomposition than from any effective invasion of particular organs.

The general symptoms of this terrible disease are: Wasting and breaking up of the system; pallor, straw-coloured tint of the skin, diarrhœa, &c.

The special symptoms depend on the organ attacked, and consist in modification of its functions or in those of neighbouring or dependent organs.

Cancer of the Tonsils.

Hindrance to swallowing and to speech produced by a large, unequal, modulated, hard tumour, sometimes bleeding, situated between the arches of the palate, are the characteristic marks of cancer of the tonsils. This kind of cancer is only met with in adults.

Cancer of the Stomach.

In cancer of the stomach, the cardiac or pyloric orifice, the larger or smaller curvatures of the organ are the seat of a morbid growth which develops in the gastric mucous membrane, extending to adjacent parts, and producing narrowing of the organ or of its orifices. Cancer of the cardiac, or entering, orifice, causes contraction of the opening, and, consequent upon this, dilatation of the œsophagus, and it causes vomiting of food soon after it has been ingested. Cancer of the pyloric, or issuing, orifice, by producing contraction of this opening, occasions considerable dilatation of the stomach, and prolonged retention of food in its cavity; it is with difficulty that it passes on into the intestines. Vomiting does not occur till two or three hours after a meal.

Scirrhus, encephaloid, epithelial cancer, or cancroid, and colloid substance in greater or less quantity, are the anatomical constituents of cancer of the stomach.

Gastralgia and pains in the back, weight at the stomach, eructations, either inodorous or sulphurous, glairy regurgitations, neutral or acid, black vomit consisting of half-digested blood—these symptoms, with a tumour felt and perceptible by touch or pressure at the epigastrium, are certain marks of cancer of the stomach. Cancer of the stomach may last for some years; but ultimately it causes death from inanition, or from peritonitis consequent on rupture, or from exhaustion, or from the cancerous cachexia with the characteristic straw-coloured tint of the face and surface.

Tumour on the Upper or Cardiac Orifice of the Stomach.

Treatment.—C. in dilution or C^5 second dilution. Baths of S^5 or C^5. Applications of R. E. alt. Y. E. to the solar plexus, or sympathetic nerve, or occiput. Compresses of W. E. at the same places. Unctions of C^5 to the pit of the stomach, and of F^2 to the hypochondria.

Cancer of the Liver.

In this case the organ is augmented in volume; there are dull, lancinating pains in the right hypochondrium, extending as far as the shoulders and right arm; dyspepsia, constipation, icterus (jaundice), ascites, and anasarca. Towards the end, diarrhœa, then the special degeneration characteristic of cancer.

Cancer in the Breast.

The glandular structure of one breast is first attacked; the other is subsequently affected as the infection spreads. Three stages are to be noted: that of formation of cancerous deposit; that of increasing growth; and that of general infection of the system with deep ulceration, numerous secondary deposits in the other breast, then in the bones, the liver, &c.

Cancer of the Spinal Cord.

In the spinal cord the indications resemble those belonging to any similar cerebral growths or tumours: that is to say, pains in the head; disordered sensation; perverted faculties; paralysis; convulsions. It is also characterized by paralysis of the lower limbs.

Cancer of the Palate.

In the palate, the cancerous tumour is diffused and has no definite outline; sometimes there is an encysted tumour, which may become as large as a pigeon's egg. Subsequently, cancer of the tongue, of the mucous lining of the pharynx, of the eye, of the bones, bringing on general disorganization and entire decomposition of the blood.

Cancer of the Lungs.

If, in a non-scrofulous adult, slight, scanty expectoration of blood occurs with oppression and some amount of feebleness in breathing; if the thoracic resonance, in percussion, is weak; if there is absence of respiratory murmur; if the echo of the voice is heard, without the attendant bronchial breeze: all these signs make the presence of pulmonary cancer to be suspected.

There is a form of cancroid disease seated in the skin, which is simply a cutaneous degeneration. It appears most frequently on the face, the lips, the neck of the uterus, the external parts of the generative apparatus, the anus, the tongue, the gullet, the stomach, the intestinal tract, the rectum. It is essentially local, and does not poison the system generally.

We can assert that Electro-Homœopathy really possesses precious agents which can neutralize the virus, and destroy the cancerous diathesis. The efficacy of the Cancerosos must astonish every careful observer. Under their administration he will see a veritable conflict between disease and remedy. And if the cancer is only in process of formation, if the tumour or ulceration is of recent occurrence, and the infection of the tissues proceeds so slowly as to allow the blood to be repaired, we shall see the cancerous disease become retrograde and then disappear. The more early the disease is taken in hand, the more rapid will be its cure.

Symptoms of Cancer.—The cancerous gland presents the following indications:—1. Hardness; more or less marked. 2. Want of sensibility to touch. 3. Tendency (i.) to enlarge, more or less slowly, after having remained stationary for years; (ii.) to become fixed after having been for a long time movable; (iii.) to adhere to the overlying skin; (iv.) to give to this skin a more or less deep-red tinge.

The open gland, the cancerous sore, has—1. Hard, raised, ragged edges. 2. Lancinating pains. 3. Black or dirty colour of the interior, which is opened. 4. Serous, limpid discharge, like water. 5. Fœtid odour.

When a cancer is retrograde it gradually loses all these characteristics, almost in the reverse order in which they had appeared. The gland becomes reduced in size, less indurated, less adherent, less discoloured; it becomes movable, it gains a certain degree of sensibility; it dwindles, dissolves, softens, and finally disappears altogether. The sore looses its fœtor, pain is diminished, and then entirely suppressed—so much so that in cancer cases treated too late we have seen the patient fade away through feebleness, but without suffering any pain. The colour passes from black to red—still later it becomes rose-tinted. Fragments of cancerous substance detach themselves and fall off at each dressing, while the margins become reduced, levelled, smoothed, and lose their sensitiveness. The suppuration is gradually changed in quality; the pus becomes creamy, thick, yellowish or slightly rose-coloured.

While this long process of constitutional clearing up is going on, we may be well assured that the medicine is operative, and we must be very careful not to change treatment in any way, and especially not to interrupt it, not even for a single day.

In some cancers, especially in the head, the lips or the uterus, the tumour may fall off in a mass instead of being broken up and disintegrated by fragments. In other cases, the cancer, apparently cured, suddenly resumes fresh activity. The treatment should then be modified, either by diminution of the dose, or by the use of other Canceroso medicines.

As the Cancerosos are the most powerful purifiers of the blood and the lymph, and as cancer rarely appears except in persons of angioitic constitution, either pure or mixed, we know that the two principal remedies are C. and A. If there is fever, F. must be added to these two until the fever is dispersed. The use of F. at the commencing and febrile crisis of absorption, is efficacious in arresting the fever, and allows the cure to proceed at an accelerated rate.

Lastly, when the cancer, after having taken visible steps in the direction of cure, is arrested, and resists the action of accustomed medicines, we are obliged to combat this inertia by administering twenty globules of C^5 in a single dose, which may be repeated for several successive days. Moreover we may resort to the use of Ver. in all obstinate cases, when the natural antidote fails; since the presence of worms of all kinds may destroy the efficacy of the remedies. Any degenerate state of the body may occasion the development of these parasites.

Under these circumstances we add to the treatment 10 globules of Ver. dry on the tongue, to be taken at bedtime; then, on waking, the first or second dilution of the same remedy, without however discontinuing C. and A. We should endeavour as far as possible to keep on with C. without any intermission, adding A. according to the proportion of vascular disorder. If C. has not produced the desired effect in the doses prescribed, or if the curative process ceases after having lasted for some time, or is not so marked as formerly, C^5 may with advantage be substituted for C^1.

As soon as the disease is subdued, treatment must yet be continued for some time, by the use of C. and subsequently of S. After a time this may be given in dry globules only.

In grave cases, and in subjects enfeebled by age, the use of S. ought to be continued during the whole remaining period of life. It is always easy to take it in the wine or beverage taken at meal-times.

Internal treatment.—For the first month the second dilution of A. alt. C. Try the first dilution as soon as the patient can bear it—using A. in the morning and C. in the afternoon. Every hour a globule of C. dry on the tongue; five globules of C. in wine or beverage at each meal. If the patient complains of indigestion or weakness, 5 globules of S. should be given dry on waking in the morning, and 2 or 3 after each meal. After the first month, if C. produces little or no effect, give C^5 alternately with A^2; 1 globule of C^5 every hour; 10 globules of C^1 in wine at meal-times.

External treatment.—Three times a day—on waking, at midday, and at bedtime—unctions of C^5 on the tumour; *i.e.* if it is not open, for we must never put greasy applications on open wounds. For the unctions glycerine may be used; it brings the remedy into closer contact with the skin.

Three time a day, unctions of A^3 to the heart, and of F^2 to the hypochrondia; and application of R. E. alt. Y. E. to the sympathetic, the solar plexus, the occiput, the pit of the stomach, and all the nerves near the tumour. On waking, 5 drops of W. E. on the skull.

We should constantly leave on the tumour, whether it is ulcerated or not, medicated compresses—renewed frequently, because when they become dry their activity ceases. If the tumour is not open, a small piece of rag soaked with R. E. should be placed on the tumour; and this should be covered with a large compress well moistened with lotion of C^5 (20 globules to the tumblerful of water); and then with a gummed cloth to keep the compresses fresh and adherent to the skin.

If the tumour is liable to hæmorrhage the rag should be moistened with B. E., and then covered with a large compress of C^5.

If the tumour is ulcerated the rag should be moistened with G. E., and covered with C5 compress. Usually full baths twice a week, lasting from fifteen to twenty minutes, according to the state of the patient. These should be of A3 and C5 alternately. In cases where the nervous system is strongly excited, a bath of F2 from time to time will give calmness.

If after long treatment a cancerous wound shows symptoms of cicatrization, this process must be accelerated by compresses of S. The internal use of S. and baths of the same should be continued for some time.

For all other kinds of cancer—whether in the eye, the uterus, or the throat—baths, compresses, gargles, injections, enemata, &c., with the remedies already indicated.

In cases of extreme suffering the dilution should be lowered for one or two days only, and the higher form resumed as soon as the suffering is abated. If doses are reduced in respect to dilution, a corresponding reduction must be made in the bath, compresses, and in fact in all external treatment. Never despair: for by perseverance we are sure to conquer. The disease may last for months, even for years; all depends on the gravity of the case. The patient should be weighed from time to time. Increase of weight is a certain sign that the tissues of the body are being repaired rather than disorganized; and however severe the suffering may be, we may rest assured that the work of reorganization will be completed.

Lupus.

A corroding eruption, serpiginous incrustations or scabs, consisting of livid and reddish spots, which, on becoming ulcerated, are liable to destroy the surrounding skin.

An acrid liquid oozes from the ulcers, and the face is covered with a greyish crust, more or less thick. It occurs mostly on the face.

Treatment.—S. in dilution alt. C., which must be alternated in obstinate cases with A., and in syphilitic subjects with Ven. The same remedies, 5 to 10 globules, dry, at meals. Alternating compresses of the same remedies. Applications of R. E. for lymphatic persons, B. for angioitic, and if there is suppuration, C. in dilution, and unctions or compresses of C^5. Towards the end S. internally and externally, which is the great agent in the cicatrization of wounds. Baths and compresses of C^5, A^2, and W. E. R. E. and Y. E. to all the sympathetic nervous centres.

Exostosis, Osteitis.

Swelling of the bone arising from scrofulous, cancerous, or syphilitic virus. Periostitis, scrofulous,or other.

Treatment.—S. in dilution, or L. alt. C^4. The same remedies at meal-time. Baths of C^5. Applications of R. E. to the sympathetic nerve. Compress of C^4. Unctions of F^2 to the hypochondria.

Syphilitic Exostosis.

Treatment.—Ven. in dilution, Alt. C^4. Baths of C^5. Applications of R. E. to the sympathetic nerve.

Necrosis

Is a term applied to the death of the whole or part of a bone. Necrosis is to the bones what gangrene is to the softer parts; the necrosed portion of bone, being dried up and deprived of its natural moisture, becomes a foreign body, analogous to a gangrenous slough.

Treatment.—C. in dilution; C^4 or C^5. Compresses with the same remedies on the diseased parts. Unctions of C^5 in the dorsal region of the spine, and if syphilitic origin is suspected, add Ven. in weak doses.

Tumours.

See Cancer, Abscess, White Swelling of the Knee or Elbow.

Special attention must be given to any tumour which is at once hard and painless; for these are marked characteristics of early cancer. In such cases we must without the least delay use the cancerous remedies both internally and externally.

Fungus Hæmatodes: Mushroom Growths.

A peculiar tumour constituted by morbid growth of the blood-vessels. Flabby growths, red, violet, or bluish, easily bleeding; in the shape of a strawberry or mushroom growing on an ulcerated surface.

Treatment.—Dil. A. alt. S. second dilution. Baths of C5 alt. A. or S5. Unctions and compresses of A2 to the heart, and of F2 to the hypochondria.

Cysts.

A formation of bags filled with serous fluid, either external or internal; in the stomach, ovaries, &c. If internal or ovarian they may exist for a long time without being suspected, until their bulk disturbs adjacent organs. These tumours easily become scirrhus or cancerous.

Treatment.—External tumours, if treated at the commencement with S. in dilution and in unctions, are easily dissipated. If they are of long standing, or internal, C1 in dilution must be used. C5 in unctions over the part where the cyst is situated, and C5 baths. Compresses of R. E. on the protuberance. A. alt. S. in dilution have succeeded in certain cases.

Indolent Glandular Tumours.

Engorgement and swelling of the glands situated under the lower jaw and down the neck. These swollen glands may also occur in the groin, the axilla, and below the hamstrings. The patients are sometimes pale, etiolated, without strength, and have diarrhœa; others, on the contrary, are fresh, and have full bodily development. Lymphatic temperaments are predisposed to this affection, which is hereditary.

Treatment.—S. in dilution alt. C. or C^5. Application of R. E. alt. Y. E. to the grand sympathetic, solar plexus, on all the neighbouring parts or those threatened, and on the tumours before they open. Baths of C^5, S., A^3, and L.

Goitre.

Enormous enlargement of the thyroid gland. This tumour, of variable form, is perforated by large veins which are often dilated and varicose.

Treatment.—C. in dilution alt. S. alt. A. second dilution. One globule of C^5 dry hourly. Compresses of W. E. and of C^5. Application of R. E. alt. Y. E. to the related nerves and all round the base of the gland.

DISEASES OF THE HEAD AND NERVOUS SYSTEM.

Pain of Various Kinds.

All occasional neuralgic or rheumatic pains generally disappear under the action of the electricities. When any pain resists electricity, the inference is that the nerves are no longer conductors, because of fixed humours or secretions obstructing the nervous currents. In this case we resort to compresses of A^2 in order to re-establish conduction, and the electricities may then be employed with good effect.

If pain returns after having disappeared, this is a proof that it proceeds from some deeper constitutional cause, and internal treatment must be added.

Aggravation of severe pain during the night indicates the presence of syphilitic virus.

Pain in the right side, extending to the dorsal spine, and fixing itself under the right shoulder-blade, indicates disorder in the liver.

Pain in the left side, attended by vertigo and palpitation, gives reason to suspect disease of the heart.

We must therefore choose the remedy according to symptoms.

If there is any point in the sternum, or breast-bone, near the clavicles or collar-bones, very sensitive to touch, it is probable that syphilitic disease exists. A sensitive or painful spot on the skull and upon the sagittal suture indicates hysterical conditions in women.

Pains in the bones of the nose, becoming worse at night, indicate hereditary syphilis lurking in the constitution.

Occasional neuralgia is dissipated at once by compresses of W. E. if the head is suffering, or of R. E. for other parts alt. Y. E. or R. E. In all cases the electricities should be first tried, by compresses or direct application; first R. E. then W. E.; then R. E. alt. Y. E. Baths and unctions of C^5, A^2, or F^2 on the painful parts. Dil. S., A^3, C^5, or F.

Congestive Neuralgia.

A. in dilution, or A. in the second dilution. Baths of A^2 or B. or W. E. Unctions and compresses of A^2 on the painful parts.

Venereal Neuralgia.

Ven. in dilution in the second dilution. Baths of Ven. alt. C^5 or S., or S^5 (100 globules). Unctions and compresses of C^5, Ven., S^5. Application of R. E. alt. Y. E. to the painful parts. Unctions of F^2 to the hypochondria.

Rheumatic Pains.

Treatment.—Dil. S. and unctions of S. alt. Ven. Application of R. E. or other electricities to the parts and the related nerve centres.

Articular (Joint) Pains.

Treatment.—Dil. A. alt. S. Baths of A. alt. C^5. Application of S. E. or B. E. Subcutaneous injection of W. E. assuages the pain.

Periosteal Pains (on the surface of Bones).

Treatment.—Dil. S. alt. C4 second dilution. Baths of C5. Compresses of C4 to the painful parts. Compresses of W. E. Application of B. E. to the sympathetic.

General Pains, over the whole Body.

Treatment.—Twenty globules of C5 dry on the tongue. Baths of S., L., C5.

Nocturnal Pains.

Treatment.—Ven. in dil. Baths of C5. Unctions of C5 or A2 on the painful part. Compresses of W. E.

Pains in the Head.

Treatment for all pains in the head. In the first place, make a light application of W. E. to the temples, the root of the nose, the sub- and super-orbital regions, the small hypoglossi, the forehead, the dorsal spine, the soles of the feet. R. E., Y. E., and B. E. may also be employed.

If the pain returns and it is supposed to be nervous, S. in small doses, alt. F. Unctions of F2 to the hypochondria. Baths of L. or S5.

If it is congestive, A3 in very small doses, then B. E. to all the nerve-points just noted.

If the pains in the head arise from uterine disorder, or leucorrhœa, C. should be given in very small doses. Unctions of C5 over the whole head. Baths of C5; 1 globule of C5 every hour.

For Migraine, and all kinds of head neuralgia returning periodically.—F. in the second dilution. Unctions of F2 or C5 to the hypochondria. *See* section on Megrim.

For exhaustion of the brain, consequent on intellectual effort.—S. dil., and in obstinate cases C. alt. S. second dilution. Headache sometimes disappears if the whole head is bathed or washed in a lotion of S., 30 globules to the quart.

Pains in the Skull.

Treatment.—Dil. C. second dilution. Baths of C^5. Unctions of C^5 to the painful part. Application of W. E. to the skull and the great sympathetic. Unctions of F^2 to the hypochondria.

Cephalalgia (Headache).

Treatment.—The same treatment, with the addition of W. E. compresses on the supra- and infra-orbital regions, and unctions of C^5 over the whole head.

Pain in the Right Side.

Treatment.—Dil. F. Unctions of F^2 to the hypochondria. Compresses of W. E.

Pain in the Left Side.

Treatment.—Dil. A. Baths of C^5. Compresses and unctions of A^2 to the heart. Application of W. E. to the sympathetic.

Pains in the Bones of the Nose.

Treatment.—Dil. Ven. second dilution. Unctions of Ven.; of C^5. Compresses of W. E.

Dental Neuralgia (Toothache).

Treatment.—Like venereal neuralgia. Also gargles of S^5, C^5, or A^3.

Pain in the Upper Part of the Sternum or Breastbone.

Treatment.—Dil. Ven. second dilution. Baths of C^5 or of S., L., or W. E. Compresses of Ven. or of C^5.

Pains in the Arms, from Injury.

Treatment.—Dil. A. alt. S. Baths of C^5, of A^2, of L. or S. Unctions and compresses of C^5 and W. E. Application of R. E. to the related nerves. Unctions of F^2 to the hypochondria.

Pains in the Knee: White Swelling.

Treatment.—Dil. C. Baths and compresses of C. or C^5. Unctions of C^5. Applications of R. E. alt. Y. E. to the related nerves.

Megrim.

Neurosis characterized by a more or less severe pain in the frontal region of the head.

Symptoms.—Loss of appetite, nausea, vomiting, red or pale face. This disorder returns at fixed periods.

Treatment.—If supposed to be nervous, S. in the second dilution, alt. with F. Unctions of C^5 over the head and neck. Light compresses of W. E. on the cranium. Application of W. E. to the occiput, small hypoglossi and sympathetic.

If congestive, A. in dilution, alt. F. the second dilution. Unctions of A^2 over the head and neck. Baths of A^2. Unctions of F^2 to the hypochondria, and of A^2 to the heart. Application of B. E. to the occiput, small hypoglossi and sympathetic.

If originating in uterine disorder or leucorrhœa, C. in the second dilution. 1 globule of C^5 every half-hour. Baths of C^5. Application of W. E. to the occiput, sympathetic, and to the soles of the feet. If the pain is periodical, F. in dilution. Unctions of F^2 to the hypochondria.

NEUROSIS GENERALLY (DISEASE OF THE NERVES).

Treatment.—S. or A. in the first dilution. Baths of C^5, or dilution of W. E. or S^5. Unctions and compresses of C^5 alt. S^5. Unctions of F^2 to the hypochondria. Application of R. E. alt. Y. E. to the occiput, sympathetic, and down each side of the dorsal spine. F. in dilution.

NERVOUS AGITATION.

Treatment.—S. in dilution, also A. and F. in the second and third dilution, with unctions of F^2 to the hypochondria. Light application of W. E. to the occiput, sympathetic, and solar plexus. For angioitic persons, compresses of A^2 to the heart. Baths of L. alt C^5.

NERVOUS CONDITIONS RESULTING FROM THE ABUSE OF QUININE.

Treatment.—S. in dilution, alt. F. in the second dilution. Baths of C^5 alt. F^2. Application of R. E. alt. Y. E. to the grand sympathetic, to the solar plexus, and occiput.

INSANITY.

All insanity unconnected with organic change can certainly be cured by the Mattei medicines.

It has been observed that in women certain disorders of the uterus may bring on insanity, in which case C. is specific, and its influence is conspicuous. Generally small doses of S. second dilution for men, and of C. for women.

GENERAL WEAKNESS OF BODY AND MIND.

Treatment.—S. in dilution, second dilution. Baths of C^5. Applications of R. E.

HYPOCHONDRIASIS.

Treatment.—C. in dilution alt. F. second dilution. Baths

of C^5. Unctions of F^2 to the hypochondria and compresses of W. E. Application of R. E. alt. Y. E. to the sympathetic nerve and solar plexus.

Violent Attacks of Mania.

Treatment.—S. in dilution, second dilution. 20 globules dry. Baths of C^5 and of W. E.

Nymphomania.

Treatment.—C. in dilution, second or third dilution Baths of C^5. Unctions of C^5 on the sacrum.

Somnambulism.

Treatment.—In women: C. Dil., or C^5 alt. F. second dilution. Baths of C^5 and of F^2. Unctions of F^2 to the hypochondria. Application of W. E. to the occiput and the great sympathetic.

In men: S. or S^5 alt. F. first dilution. Unctions of F^2 to the hypochondria. Baths of S^5 and of L.

Hysteria: Neurosis.

A disease, as a rule, only occurring in women, in which there is excessive nervous irritability, commencing with uneasiness, cramps, spasms, marked change of character, fantastic dreams, then the sensation of a ball which seems to rise in the chest and provoke a crisis (the globus hystericus); pain shooting through the sagittal suture or centre line of the skull (hysterical clavus), pain in the back on any pressure on the stomach, pain in the joints; convulsive movements, nervous paroxysms, tears, screams, sadness, hallucinations; faculty of distinguishing people simply by the smell, hearing at a considerable distance, fear of any noise, scents, perfumes—as soon as the meat is cut appetite goes; persistent smelling of an imaginary odour; purely fanciful oppression; everything imaginative; thirst; frequent and almost colourless urine; hysterical cough, sometimes barking, cold in the extremities, the face quickly flushing and heating. All this group of phenomena are generally due to some disorder of the uterus, either local uterine disease, or sexual privation, or the reverse, excess. Hysteria has often led to mental alienation and epilepsy; it is rarely fatal, and can be cured.

Treatment.—C^1 in dilution, or S^1 alt. A^3 if the temperament is of a pronounced angioitic type. Four teaspoonfuls of the second or third glass every day. The dose should be extremely weak if the disease is to be diminished and not augmented. For clavus hystericus, lotion of W. E. on the painful part. Hysterical crises are often cut short by B. E. applied to the pit of the stomach.

Encephalitus.

Inflammation of the substance of the brain. This disease is rarer and less understood than inflammation of the meninges or covering membranes. The symptoms are very similar, viz.: Fever, insomnia, intense headache, difficulty in bearing light, delirium, somnolence, coma.

Treatment.—S. in the second dilution; if necessary, C., alt. A^3. Compresses all over the head of W.E., C^5, B.E. Unctions of F^2 on the hypochondria.

Meningitis.

Inflammation of the coverings of the brain. A very grave disease, and sometimes difficult to diagnose.

Symptoms.—Violent headache, sleepiness, insomnia, intense fever, vomitings and constipation; then delirium, convulsions, intolerance of noise, light, and movement, comatose sleep. Afterwards, all these acute symptoms give place to profound stupor; the face is pale, expression of face stupid, vital heat diminishes, and death ensues.

Treatment.—C. or S. in the second dilution. Moisten the head lightly with W. E. Unctions or compresses of C., S., A^2, or B. E., on the head. Application of R. E. to the smaller hypoglossi. Application of R E. alt. Y. E. to the occiput, temples, and sympathetic.

Apoplexy.

Is sometimes preceded by vertigo, dazzling, heaviness in the head.

Symptoms.—Effusion of blood, more or less extensive, in the brain, producing partial or complete loss of consciousness, with loss of sensation or motor power in one or more portions of the body. Effusion of blood in the brain and lungs, and serous infiltration in the cranial and cerebral cells, are the causes.

Treatment.—We begin in all cases by giving 8 or 10 globules, dry, of S.; and this dose should be repeated every ten minutes till digestive functions are restored, for in almost all cases this attack is complicated by an arrest of digestive function.

Sanguineous Apoplexy.

Very weak doses of A. third dilution. Application of B. E. to all the central points. Compresses of A. or A^2 (20 globules to a glass of water). Application of W. E. to the seat of effusion.

Serous Apoplexy.

Treatment.—S. dry, 10 or 20 globules at the outset of the attack if it is hidden; repeat this, if necessary, after a quarter of an hour. Dil. S. second or third dilution.

Softening of the Brain.

This usually arises after attacks of congestion of the brain. The principal symptoms are pale face, heavy and stupid air (hebetude), failure in intellect, semi-paralysis or hemiplegia, sometimes imbecility.

Treatment.—Dil. C. alt. S. alt. A. The same remedies at meals. 1 globule of C^5 every half-hour. Baths of C^5 alt. A^2 alt. S., or of W. E., R. E., or B. E. Unctions of C^5 alt. A^3 alt. S^5 over the head. Unctions of F^2 to the hypochondria.

Vertigo (Giddiness).

Treatment.—According to temperament. S. or A., sometimes F. After miscarriage, if there is vertigo, give C. in very small doses. Unctions of F^2 or C^5 to the hypochondria.

Coma.

Drowsiness more or less deep, from which it is difficult to rouse the patient. Indications of vascular congestion, or of some effusion into the cavities of the brain. This symptom is observed in meningitis and in all cerebral disorders.

Treatment.—Dil. S. in small doses, with R. E. If the lethargy is congestive, A. in very small doses, and unctions of A^2 over the heart.

Convulsions.

Convulsive movements of the body; trismus, or lock-jaw; clenching of the teeth; abolition more or less complete of sensation and consciousness. It attacks young children, and women—often after or during confinement.

Treatment.—Dil. S. second dilution. Unctions of C^5 or S^2 on the jaws. Application of Y. E. to the occiput, the great sympathetic, and on the jaws.

Spasms, or Cramp.

Convulsive contractions of the muscles, variously situated.

Treatment.—If they arise from worms, Ver. dil. or $Ver.^2$ second dilution. Baths of W. E. or C^5. If they do not arise from worms, they will disappear with S. or C. in small and reduced doses. Baths of L.

CONTRACTIONS.

Nervous contractions in all parts of the body.

Treatment.—Are ordinarily dissipated by R. E. to the sympathetic, occiput, and solar plexus. Baths of C5, which may be alternated with baths of W. E. or of L. Application of W. E. over the skull.

PERIODIC OR CHRONIC SPASMS.

Dil. S. Application of R. E. to the sympathetic, solar plexus, occiput, along the dorsal spine on each side.

At the menstrual period.—Dil. A. and compresses of A. over the heart and of B. E. to the stomach. However, for lymphatics S. is to be preferred.

In the legs.—Cramps in the extremities disappear with unctions and compresses of C5, Dil. S.; and, if necessary, compresses of W. E.

In the hands.—Unctions of C5 and compresses of W. E. 10 globules of S. dry on the tongue. Application of R. E. to the wrist and the whole length of the thumb.

At the nape of the neck.—10 globules, dry, of S. Unctions of L. or of C5. Application of R. E. alt. Y. E. to the nape.

At the eyelids.—Dil. S. Application of R. E. to the supra- and infra-orbital nerves.

At the heel: the tendon Achilles.—Application of R. E. to the nerves of the leg, especially the ankles. In obstinate cases, unctions of C5. Baths of C5, and Dil. S.

TRISMUS (LOCK-JAW).

Partial tetanus, consisting in spasmodic closure of the jaws.

Treatment.—At first apply Y. E. or R. E. alt. Y. E. to the cheek and occiput; if this is not sufficient, it should be applied to the sympathetic; and if by these remedies the nerves are not released, add S. internally. Compresses of C5 and W. E. on the jaws. Baths of C5 and of L.

SHOCKS, STROKE, LIGHTNING, ETC.

Treatment.—10 globules of S. dry. Applications of R. E. alt. Y. E. to the solar plexus, occiput, grand sympathetic, and all the nerves of the head. Compresses of W. E. over the head.

INSOLATION (SUNSTROKE).

Treatment.—S. in dilution alt. A3 first dilution. 1 globule of C5 every half-hour. Baths of C5. Unctions of C5 over the head. Compresses of W. E. Application of R. E. alt. Y. E. to the occiput, sympathetic, sub and supra orbital regions, forehead, and temples.

INTOXICATION.

Treatment.—10 grains of S. dry, all at once, on the tongue. After one hour repeat, in order to overcome it entirely.

INTOXICATION AND ITS CONSEQUENCES.

Treatment.—S. in dilution, first dilution, or A. (second dilution). 20 globules of C5 each day. Unctions of F2 to the hypochondria, of A. on the heart. Baths of C5. Application of W. E. to the sympathetic and solar plexus.

DELIRIUM TREMENS.

Treatment.—Dil. S. second dilution. Baths of L. Application of W. E. to the skull and along the dorsal spine.

HYDROCEPHALUS.

An infantine disease, depending upon a large effusion of serum in the interior and exterior of the brain, in the ventricles, or in the arachnoid cavity.

With adults, serum is sometimes deposited in the meninges or in the cerebral substance, but this is rather serous effusion or œdema than true hydrocephalus.

Hydrocephalus is recognized by an excessive and regular development of the cranium, the volume of which is greatly enlarged in comparison to the dimensions of the face, the soft, fibrous walls of which gradually lose their bony constituents. The size of the head is sometimes such that the children, unable to bear the weight, are obliged to remain in bed, and the soft cranium flattens and is deformed by the pressure of the pillow.

The cranium of children attacked by hydrocephalus has a circumference varying from two to five feet.

There is an enormous quantity of clear, liquid serum, containing a very small proportion of salines or albumen, composed of 99 parts of water in every 100 (Marcet), deposited in the lateral ventricles or in the arachnoid cavity. This it is which causes the development of the cranium in patients attacked with hydrocephalus.

Arachnoid hydrocephalus often results from a meningeal hæmorrhage, which is absorbed and is transformed into a serous cyst, which invades the substance of the brain, and possibly drives it back on to the base of the cranium. Ventricular hydrocephalus sometimes dilates the ventricles, converting the cerebral hemispheres into two pockets in juxtaposition, the upper walls of which are only about a quarter of an inch thick; but it will be understood that the patient, before arriving at this stage, may show much variety in the degrees of development. A child suddenly attacked with convulsions, and who has developed chronic hydrocephalus after several months, has probably arachnoid hydrocephalus, following upon a meningeal hæmorrhage. (Legendre.)

Hydrocephalus generally brings on paralysis of the limbs and organs of sense in children; sight is weak, and the eyes divergent, the pupils are dilated and are continually oscillating. Hearing and smell are abolished; speech is slow or absent; walking is unsteady or impossible; digestion remains good, but the evacuations are involuntary, and often there are vomitings or convulsions, which are provoked by movement or by any pressure on the cranium. (Despiès.)

Treatment.—C. in dilution alt. A. second or third dilution. Baths and unctions over the whole head of C5. Compresses of B. E. on the cranium. Application of Y. E. to the grand sympathetic, solar plexus, occiput, and all the nerves of the head. Unctions of F^2 to the hypochondria.

PARALYSIS.

It is amenable to treatment when sudden or accidental, provoked by drink, &c.

Treatment.—20 or 25 globules of S. dry, in one dose, or bathe the head with W. E. Application of R. E. alt. Y. E. to the occiput, sympathetic, and solar plexus. Unctions and compresses to the head of C5 or S.

THREATENING OF GENERAL PARALYSIS.

Treatment.—Application of R. E. to the sympathetic and solar plexus, and especially to the pit of the stomach. If there is vascular congestion, A. in dilution or A^2 in the second dilution. The same remedies dry, 5 globules alternately at meal-times. Compresses of A^2 on the heart. Baths of A^2. Continue this treatment until a cure is effected.

NERVOUS PARALYSIS.

Without angioitic indications.

Treatment.—S. in dilution alt. C5. The same remedies dry alt., 5 globules at meal-times. Moisten the head with W. E. Application of R. E. alt. Y. E. to the occiput, sympathetic, solar plexus, and all the nerves of the head. Baths of S., C5, or W. E.

VASCULAR PARALYSIS.

Treatment.—A. in the second dilution. 5 globules of A^2, dry, twice a day. Compresses of A^2 to the heart and B. E. to the head. Unctions of F^2 or C^5 to the hypochondria. Baths of B. E., 2 or 3 tablespoonfuls to a bath.

Nervous Paralysis of the Tongue.

Treatment.—S. in the first dilution. 10 globules of S. in wine at each meal. Gargles of S. alt. C^5. Application of R. E. to the large and small hypoglossi, occiput, and sympathetic. Baths of C^5 alt. S. and R. E. (3 tablespoonfuls to a bath).

Vascular Paralysis of the Tongue.

Treatment.—A^3 in the second dilution. 5 globules of A^3, dry, twice a day. Gargles of A^3 alt. B. E. Baths of A^3. Application of B. E. to the large and small hypoglossi.

Paralysis of the Prostrate or of the Bladder, consequent on Hypertrophy of the Prostrate.

Treatment.—S. in dilution alt. A^3. 5 globules C^5, dry, twice a day. Sitz baths of tepid water medicated with 50 globules of S^5 or C^5. Application of W. E. to the pubes, the sacrum, and the perinæum. Baths of W. E. (3 tablespoonfuls to a bath).

General Paralysis.

Consequent on hæmorrhagic apoplexy, sometimes with varicose ulcers on the legs and general plethora.

A. in dilution, A^2 first dilution, 10 globules in the wine at meal-time. Baths, unctions, and compresses of A^3 alt. C^5. Application of B. E. in compresses on all the nerves of the head, and down the dorsal spine. Unctions of F^2 or C^5 on the hypochondria. Compresses on the heart of A^3 (4 globules to a tablespoonful of water).

Paralysis of the Generative System.

Treatment.—First dilution of S. alt. A. The same

remedies dry at meal-time. Unctions of C5 and S., S2 on the paralyzed parts. Baths of C. alt. S. alt. A. alt. W. E. or B. E. Application of R. E. alt. Y. E. to the sacrum, perinæum, and pubes.

Dumbness (Mutism).

Loss of speech. Almost always cured by the electricities alone. The choice of the electricity must depend on the temperament of the patient.

Treatment.—S. in the second dilution, C. in the second dilution, A2 in the second dilution. Unctions to the whole of the head with C5 or S5. Unctions or compresses of F2 to the hypochondria. Application of R. E. alt. Y. E. to the hypoglossi, occiput, and sympathetic. Baths of L. and W. E. (3 spoonfuls of electricity in a bath).

Stammering.

This conditon may be habitual or casual; it sometimes occurs in nervous fevers.

Treatment.—Application of R. E. to the great and little hypoglossi, Dil. S. Gargles of R. E. or W. E. Baths of L., C5, or A2.

Insomnia.

Want of sleep. This phenomenon may exist by itself and constitute a veritable disease, or be connected with some other disorder. The principal causes producing insomnia are pain, continual wish to change position or to pass off any secretion, cough, dyspnœa, agitation of the mind; sometimes prolonged watching ends in producing obstinate insomnia.

Treatment.—S. in dilution, first dilution. 1 globule of C5 every half-hour. Unctions of F2 to the hypochondria, grand sympathetic, and solar plexus. Application of R. E. alt. Y. E. to all the nerves of the head. Moisten the head slightly with W. E. If the insomnia is the result of a febrile condition of the blood, 3 or 4 spoonfuls of F[1], second dilution, will dissipate it. 2 globules of S., repeated every quarter of an hour, has been found successful.

Epilepsy.

A non-febrile, non-inflammatory, chronic, and intermittent affection of the brain, taking the form of fits.

These fits or attacks, when the disease has reached a certain point, are characterized by general or partial convulsions, loss of intelligence, insensibility of all parts of the body, but without consecutive paralysis of movement or sensation. In the immense majority of cases, epileptic attacks are not preceded by premonitory symptoms. Generally at some time when the patient is not expecting any seizure he loses consciousness and falls, the eyes open wide, the pupils are fixed, the direction of the eyes is changed, the face drawn on one side, the mouth drawn towards the ear, and the teeth clenched; then, after several moments, the muscles of the neck stiffen, the head is twisted, the jugular veins swell, the face is in a state of violent turgescence, the muscles of the face undergo violent and frequent spasmodic contractions, foam forms on the lips; the upper and lower limbs, especially the former, are shaken by convulsive shocks; the thumbs are clenched. The thorax, however, remains firm and immovable, respiration is almost suspended, or superficial and irregular, and suffocation seems imminent.

This condition, which lasts from two to eight minutes, but may last much longer, and occurs at close intervals, is followed by general relaxation of the muscular system, a pale face, and gradual return of free breathing; the countenance retains for some time an air of hebetude; the intellectual and sensitive faculties, plunged in stupor, regain their activity little by little, and the patient feels a quivering of returning life in his body.

But epileptic attacks are not always so violent; sometimes there is only a quite momentary loss of consciousness, with slight and partial convulsions of the eyes, the mouth, an arm, or a finger, accompanied or not with falling. Sometimes the attack is simply a feeling of giddiness, and the patient does not lose consciousness. Finally, in some cases, the attack is preceded by a cool sensation, shivering, congestion, formication, or even pain, in some part either close to or far from the brain, as the neck, breast, arm, foot, &c., and from this place there comes a singular sensation like a stream or *aura*, travelling towards the brain and provoking the phenomena which I have described. The return of the attacks occurs at greater or lesser intervals.

Some epileptics have several attacks a day, others only one. With the majority they only take place at longer intervals, and altogether very irregularly. When the disease has lasted some time, it is noticed, between the attacks, that certain disorders show themselves which indicate a more or less profound lesion of the cerebral nervous centres. Epileptics have generally obstinate, uneven dispositions; they become absent-minded, the memory and active mental faculties become weakened, and they are unable to sustain continuous exertion. These are the most favourable cases. Others become idiots; almost all, if they live long enough, fall into a state of incurable mania or insanity. Memory is the sense which is first touched. Voluntary movements also assume permanently abnormal conditions; squinting, convulsive twitches, contractions, muscular atrophy, contortions of the head, disfigurement of the face, are often developed. Otherwise, and this in great contrast to the condition of the brain, the ordinary functions of the organs of vegetative life are generally carried on with regularity.

Epilepsy occurs much more often before than after puberty. It has been observed during the first days of life, is rare in old people, and twice as frequent in women as in men. It is also more common in cold than warm countries. It is sometimes hereditary. Amongst the determining causes fright is the most frequent; this cause is especially likely to produce epilepsy when it happens to women at the monthly period. After fright, this nervous disease is most often produced through strong passions, as anger, jealousy, anxiety. Finally, epilepsy often accompanies idiotcy, and it is estimated that there is one epileptic in every eight idiots.

Few diseases are so grave as epilepsy, and it is all the more serious where it shows itself in early life and from the influence of hereditary taint; when it is accompanied by vertigo, or loss of consciousness; and when the attacks are more frequent and leave great confusion in the intellectual faculties. Sudden death occurs occasionally in very violent attacks, the result of cerebral congestion.

It is less terrible when the disease arises from a specific cause, as syphilis; or an accidental cause, as fright; when the attacks are infrequent, and the disease advances slowly. Pathological anatomy tells us nothing of the probable causes of epilepsy. The structural changes which have been found in epileptics who have succumbed to the disease, have nothing in them peculiar or characteristic. Casauviell and Bouchet say that traces of chronic inflammation of the white substance of the brain are constantly present. But even if this be admitted, it would remain to be proved whether the inflammation is not rather the effect of the congestion produced by the attack, than the cause itself of the attacks. None of the different lesions, such as intra-cranial tumours of various kinds, hydatids, effusion, alteration of the membranes, thickening or alteration in form of the cranial bones, hypertrophy, or altered structure of the brain tissue, &c., which are seen in epileptics, can be considered as peculiar to this disease. Besides, it is not easy to understand how such different changes, occurring in such entirely different parts of the encephalon, could produce such a characteristic disease, and one so uniform in its symptoms, as epilepsy.

Traumatic Epilepsy.

This is a disease characterized, like spontaneous epilepsy, by general convulsions and by complete loss of consciousness, but only of a passing nature like the causes which produce it.

Treatment.—It must be ascertained whether the patient is lymphatic or angioitic. There may be cases in which the patient suffers from worms. S. in dilution or A3 in very weak doses, second or third dilution. Baths of A2 alt. L. In case of worms Ver. The Canceroso remedies may be tried for cases in women, and if there are any signs of hysteria.

Hydrophobia (Rabies).

Rabies, or hydrophobia, is a malignant disease which is caused by the bite of a rabid animal. There is no known instance of the spontaneous occurrence in man of this disease; it is always derived from the bite of a previously infected animal. The active principle of rabies is to be found, according to some authorities, exclusively in the saliva; according to others, in the bronchial mucus. The person thus inoculated by the bite of a rabid animal does not immediately show the presence of the characteristic symptoms. A period of thirty or forty days usually elapses before the commencement of symptoms. However, this incubation period varies in different cases, it may be shorter or longer—even ten or twelve months.

The earliest symptoms are headache and insomnia; most patients are restless and depressed; others are lively and loquacious: in all cases, appetite is diminished and the pulse accelerated. These various kinds of discomfort, which may last for some days, belong to the second stage—that of prodromata. The third and final stage is first indicated by a sense of constriction and suffocation in the throat, and a dread or horror of liquids. The countenance and general appearance of the patient manifests the greatest possible terror at the sight of water, or the offer of drink. They are also painfully sensitive to any draught, to bright light, or the sight of objects having any brilliant colouring. Nevertheless, they are tormented by excessive thirst, and when, in order to assuage it, they attempt to conquer their horror of drink, they seize the cup which contains the fluid with a sort of trembling rage, bring it to their lips, and then immediately thrust it aside in fright, with the utmost dread of suffocation. Hearing is exalted; the sense of touch is heightened; speech is abrupt; some are furious, but this is not usual. As the fatal result approaches, convulsions become more and more frequent, and difficulty of respiration increases. Expectoration is continual, dark circles surround the eyes, the lips and fingers are livid; finally life ceases suddenly, without pain, by the closure of the respiratory organs. The duration of this last stage is generally two or three days.

Cases of spontaneous development of this disease have only been observed in animals belonging to the genus *canis* or *felis*, especially the dog, the wolf, the fox, and the cat.

If a dog is about to develop this terrible disease, the first indication is depression and loss of appetite. Very soon he forsakes his master's house and runs, with lowered head, furry coat standing on end, his lips covered with foaming drivel, biting all he meets, whether men or animals, without appearing to pursue them. In this animal, horror of water is a less constant symptom than in man. From time to time convulsions arise and arrest the progress of the animal; at last death comes suddenly. The dog is also subject to a modified description of rabies, *dumb rage*—dumb, that is to say, because he cannot cry. It is also equally impossible for him to bite, for he cannot open or shut his jaws. Such an animal suffers from intense anxiety, without any paroxysm of fury. Dumb rage is often, it is thought, produced by the bite of a rabid animal, but it is doubtful whether it is transmissible by inoculation.

Treatment.—1 globule, dry, of S. every ten minutes; 5 globules, dry, of F. night and morning. Unctions of F^2 to the hypochondria. Application of Y. E. to the throat and neck; of B. E. to the heart; and of W. E. on the skull, the great sympathetic, the solar plexus, and the pit of the stomach.

Alopecia, or Baldness.

Falling of the hair, arising from constitutional causes.

Treatment.—Dil. S. Unctions on the head of C^5. Application of R. E. and B. E.

Syphilitic Alopecia.—Syphilis often produces loss of hair, especially on the scalp, in either sex.

Alopecia of the scalp is an accident concerning which there is certain misapprehension prevalent, which ought to be corrected. It is, moreover, a symptom which may occur in a great variety of diseases.

It is a common opinion that alopecia is an indication of long-established venereal disorder—of disease that has existed for years in the system. If, for example, a man becomes bald when he reaches middle age, it is usual to attribute this *calvities* to "youthful follies"—that is to say, if a man of forty becomes bald, this results from disease contracted when he was a young man, fifteen or twenty years previously. Nothing can be more false than this. Baldness, so far from being a remote result of venereal disorder, is, on the contrary, one of its earliest manifestations; it is characteristic of the early months, or at most of disease dating from one or two years. It is essentially a *secondary* symptom. If its appearance is delayed longer, this is almost invariably due to the action of specific medicine which postpones and modifies the disease. After the first years of constitutional disease, that is to say, after the period of secondary disease, this type of alopecia does not occur.

Syphilitic baldness occurs in one of two ways :—

1. Either the hair falls as the result of disease of the scalp itself affecting the hair follicles ; or

2. More frequently the loss of hair occurs without any local lesion to account for it, from constitutional conditions.

In the first case it is not uncommon to find superficial ulcerative skin disease, more or less extended and confluent, more or less obstinate also in its duration. In any case, this disease causes loss of hair by alteration and disorder of the hair-bulbs.

Among the lesions of the scalp which may produce partial or diffused alopecia, of intensity proportionate to the completeness with which the eruption has taken possession of the surface, we may specify syphilitic acne, which is very common at the outset of secondary symptoms, characterized by small slightly elevated crusts, about the size of a pin's head, of a yellowish or brown tint; the papulous encrusted variety—impetigo—diffused or superficial ecthyma.

There is another variety much less known, but not less frequent, especially in women. It is allied to pityriasis, a bran-like eruption of the scalp, and consists of scattered red patches, lenticular or diffused, so pale as generally to escape observation, covered with a fine powdery desquamation, almost microscopic, and only capable of being detected by a skilled observer.

In another case, the hair falls without assignable reason, or at any rate if lesions exist they are not serious enough to account for the result; for they may explain the fall of hair in the locus of attack, but they do not explain the general loss of hair all over the head and where no special lesion is to be detected.

Syphilitic alopecia is always only temporary; it exists for a time, sometimes for weeks, more usually for months, for a year or more. Afterwards the course is invariably as follows: the lost hair reappears, the denuded surfaces are re-covered, and ultimately the scalp regains its normal state—unless, it must be observed, the injury and ulceration have been so profound as to have actually destroyed the structure of the skin; otherwise venereal disease never produces baldness.

Treatment.—In order to meet the constitutional state, Ven. in dilution, alt. C. Unctions of Ven. Baths of Ven., A., C5.

DISEASES OF THE EYES.

EYES.

Diseases of the eyes, with impaired vision.

Treatment.—All the caustics ordinarily used must be discarded. Treatment should begin with the electricities, R. E., B. E., or W. E., which, if applied to the occiput or sympathetic, or the sub- and supra-orbital regions, have a powerful effect. For in almost all cases lachrymal secretion is restored; redness diminishes, as well as the smarting, burning, and inflammation. It is important to treat both eyes at the same time and similarly, even if only one is affected.

If the disease resists the action of the electricities, internal treatment, according to the constitution of the patient, sanguine, lymphatic or mixed, must be resorted to.

Employ also eye-washes by means of a special collyrium glass, which fits the eye and can be filled with the medicated water. The strength should be 2 or 3 globules to each collyrium glass. In this way the medicine can be brought into contact with the surface of the eye-ball.

Marina, a new medicine, is found to be specific in most eye cases, and may be used instead of, or in alternation with, the above remedies.

Amblyopia.

Enfeeblement of sight.

Treatment.—A. Dil. alt. S. The same remedies at meals. 1 globule of C5 every half-hour. Baths of C5, or of S., or of A^2, or of W. E. Compresses of C5 or W. E. to the head. Application of R. E. alt. Y. E. to the occiput, sympathetic, sub- and supra-orbitals, root of the nose and frontal region. (*See* Cataract.)

Staphyloma.

A transparent or opaque tumour, formed either on the cornea or on the iris: it has the form of a grape seed.

Treatment.—Dil. S., A3. Continuous compresses, even through the night, of L., B. E., W. E., or R. E.

Ophthalmia.

Inflammation of the globe of the eye and of the mucous membrane lining the inner surface of the eyelids, and uniting them to the ball of the eye; feeling as if sand were under the eyelids, redness of the eyelids with smarting, continuous lachrymation, headache, fear of a strong light.

Treatment.—Application of R. E. or B. E. according to the constitution of the patient, to the occiput, the sub- and supra-orbital regions. S. in dilution, alt. A. in the first dilution; 1 globule of C5 dry every hour. Compresses over the head of W. E. alt. C5. Baths of C5. 10 globules of A. in the wine in the middle of the day; 10 globules of S. at dinner.

Chronic Catarrhal Ophthalmia.

Same symptoms, painless, with abundant flow of purulent serum. Same treatment.

Syphilitic Ophthalmia.

Symptoms.—Swollen and red eyelids, with thick discharge, grey spots on some parts of the eye, or covering it entirely; falling of the lashes, sometimes swelling of the glands under the jaw, yellow tint of the skin, terrified expression, with swollen or puffy face; flushed face. (*See* the chapter on Venereal Diseases.)

Lachrymation

Morbid and continuous flow of tears.

Treatment.—Bathe the eyes with R. E. Compresses of the same on the occiput. S. in dilution alt. C.

Photophobia.

A state in which light is insupportable.

Treatment.—Sometimes one single application of R. E. is sufficient,—to the occiput, sympathetic, and sub- and supra-orbitals. Or else R. E. alt. Y. E. to the same points. Compresses of W. E. and unctions of C^5 over the whole head.

Amaurosis.

Enfeeblement or total loss of sight, supervening without any apparent injury or alteration of structure in the eye itself, and without the existence of any impediment to the passage of the rays of light to the optic nerve. It is really a paralysis of the retina or optic nerve.

Treatment.—S^2 Dil., and compresses of the same to the eyes; application of W. E. or B. E. to the centre or back of the skull, to the occiput and sympathetic.

At Rome, in the hospital of Saint Theresa, as reported in Professor Pascucci's book, a case of amaurosis was overcome in one hour by applications of R. E. to the occiput.

Diplopia.

Double sight—seeing double: visual disturbance in which two distinct sensations are produced by the same object, so that everything looks double.

This disorder is mostly observed in nervous or hypochondriacal persons—in those who have suffered from great mental distress or annoyance, or in persons whose eyes have been exposed to vivid tests of endurance; or in pregnant women.

Generally diplopia is symptomatic of strasbismus or squinting; the attack is often sudden, and the patient does not always recognize at first the false sensation of which he is the subject: he thinks that there are two objects before him as he sees them. It is impossible for him to distinguish very small or very near objects—to read print, for instance.

Treatment.—Application of R. E. alt. Y. E. to the occiput, the sympathetic, the sub- and supra-orbital regions. Compresses of G. E. over the eyes. A. in dil. or S. alt. A.

Inflammation of the Eyelids.

Treatment.—S. in dilution alt. C. second dilution. The same remedies dry, 5 globules alt. twice a day. Compresses to the eyes of S., A., W. E., or C5. Application of R. E. alt. Y. E. to the occiput, sympathetic, sub- and supra-orbital regions, forehead, and root of the nose.

DISEASES OF THE EARS.

Pains in the Ears (Otalgia).

Treatment.—S. in dilution or S5 alt C., alt A^2 in the second dilution. Same remedies in wine at meal-times. Unctions and compresses of C5, S., A^2, over the ear. Application of R. E. alt. Y. E. to the small muscles behind the ear, and the hollow under the ear formed by opening the jaws. Baths of C5 alt. S., alt. A^2. Injections of W. E. (one spoonful of electricity and two of water).

Otitis and Otorrhœa.

Treated in the same manner.

For otorrhœa with toothache, add gargles of C5 or A3.

Deafness.

Treatment.—If the cause is nervous, S. dil., alt. C5 first dilution. The same remedies at meals, 5 or 10 globules. Unctions over the whole external ear of C5 or S. Compresses of W. E. frequently, to the nape of the neck and behind the ears. Injections of C5 into the ear passage.

If the cause is congestive, in a sanguine temperament, A. or A3 first dilution. Unctions and compresses of A2 over the ear. B. E. to all the nerves of the ear. Unctions of A2 over the heart. Cures have been numerous.

Buzzing in the Ears.

Treatment.—Like otalgia.

Hæmorrhage from the Ear.

Treatment.—A. in dilution, A2 in the second dilution. Compresses of A. or A2 on the heart. Application of B. E. to the occiput and sympathetic. Baths and compresses on the head with A2.

Polypus in the Ear Passages.

Treatment.—C. in the second dilution. W. E. in the ear (on a little cotton wool). One globule of C5 every half-hour. Compresses, unctions, and injections of C5 in the ear. Application of R. E. to the small muscles behind the ear. Injection of C5.

Mumps.

Inflammation of the salivary glands under the ears.

Treatment.—C. in the second dilution, C5 first dilution. One globule of C5, dry, every half-hour. Unctions and compresses of C^5 to the part. Baths of C^5. Unctions of C^5 to the hypochondria. Application of R. E. alt. Y. E. all round the tumour, repeated several times a day. Try L., at the same time five drops of W. E. on the cranium. Application of B. E. to the nape of the neck.

DISEASES OF THE NOSE.

Smell.

Loss or perversion of smell.

Treatment.—S. in dilution in the first dilution. Aspirations of the same (20 globules to a glass of water) Application of R. E. alt Y. E. to the root of the nose. Baths of C^5 to the root of the nose. Baths of C^5. Unctions and compresses of C^5, alt S., A^2, to the root of the nose.

Epistaxis: Bleeding at the Nose.

Treatment.—Dil. A^3: the doses very small, and constantly reduced if the bleeding is obstinate. Compresses of A. (10 or 15 globules to the glass) on the forehead, the nose, and the nape of the neck. Compresses of B. E. over the arteries in the neck. Inhalation of the same remedy is unfailing. In obstinate cases Dil. A^2 alt. C^5 first dilution. Inhalation of the same remedies. Application of B. E. to the root of the nose, the occiput, the sympathetic, the forehead. Unctions and compresses of A^2 on the heart.

It must be remembered that too strong doses increase hæmorrhage.

Coryza.

Cold in the head; inflammation of the lining mucous membrane of the nasal fossæ.

Symptoms.—Stoppage of the nose, eyes red, headache, hot skin.

Treatment.—Dil S., a teaspoonful every five minutes for half an hour, or some dry globules of L. on the tongue.

Unctions of C5 over the head. Application of R. E. alt. Y. E. or B. E. to the occiput and sympathetic.

Ozæna.

Fœtid exhalations from the nose are the characteristic signs of ozæna. This horrible disease has its roots in the depths of the organism; it originates in, it is developed and perpetuated by, certain constitutional germs, which differ from one another in nature, but in the evil influence which they exercise on the organism resemble the action of other malignant diseases. It can exist with or without destructive external action. The lesions which it produces are represented by ulceration of the pituitary membrane, which are variable in form, seat, and extent; whether deep or superficial, they attack the submucous cellular tissue, and even the periosteum of the bones which form the nasal fossæ. Accordingly we find caries and necrosis of the bones or cartilages, which provoke active diseases which ultimately lead to the destruction, or at least to the deformity, of the nose. When ozæna occurs with these organic changes, one is inclined to believe that the strong fœtor is due to the anatomical state of the parts by the composition of particular secretions. But this illusion does not last long. In fact ozæna may exist independently of all external lesion, and sometimes even without the slightest symptoms of coryza. It is then impossible to say whence the offensive odour, which sometimes constitutes the sole symptom of the disease, proceeds from. It has been attributed to the closure of the nasal fossæ, complicated by a vice of constitution; or it may be regarded as resulting from an accidental malformation of the nose hindering the evacuation of mucous secretions. The prolonged detention of this secretion might cause the disagreeable smell. This interpretation is not based on any serious grounds; ozæna exists independently of all banormal modification in the form of the nasal fossæ, and were this modification to exist in subjects affected by ozæna it would be necessarily anterior to the fœtor of disease. Why should we not frankly admit that we do not know the origin of ozæna? Should we hesitate to avow our limited knowledge in presence of this inexplicable phenomenon, when we find it difficult to explain the ultimate origin of disagreeable smells from the perspiration of the feet, hands, and armpits? There is some change in the functions of the organism, and this is all we can say.

This disease, which has baffled all the means ordinarily taken to alleviate it, has found in our experimental therapeutics agents of incontestible efficacy. It is easy to understand that ozæna, originating in a morbid constitutional principle, can only be radically cured by the aid of remedies possessing a general action on the organism.

Experiments have been made, and crowned with success. We shall give, amongst other cures, those effected by Dr. William J. Flogg, of New York. It is one more page to add to the golden records of Electro-Homœopathy.

Treatment.—S. in the first dilution, also S. alternately with A3 in the first dilution. Aspirations of S5, C5 (25 globules to every glassful of slightly alcoholized water). Whole baths of C5, S5, L. Unctions of C5 to the root of the nose. Application of R. E. alt. Y. E. to the root of the nose, occiput, and temples. W. E. on the cranium.

DISEASES OF THE MOUTH AND THROAT.

Stornatitis: Gangrene in the mouth.

This affection may follow acute or chronic attacks in children, commencing by aphthæ or by a small grey ulceration found on the mucous membrane of the mouth, on the inner surface of the lips, the cheek, or at the base of the gums. Later on a shining livid swelling with a hard central kernel, having a black surface, surrounded with a grey-coloured margin, granulated and bleeding; a fœtid odour, with sometimes a constant running of saliva; the skin not hot, and the pulse not accelerated.

The same treatment as the preceding; and gargles of C5, alt. A3; for children, smaller doses.

Stomatitis.—Inflammation of the mucous membrane of the mouth.

Treatment.—Dil. S. Gargle of R. E. or W. E., or of S. alt. C. Application of R. E. to the stomach. Baths of A2 or C5.

Mercurial Stomatitis.

Same treatment.

Syphilitic Stomatitis.

Dil. Ven. or S. alt. Ven. Gargle with the same medicines. Application of R. E. to the pit of the stomach. In obstinate cases, give C5, one globule every hour, and C5 in dilution.

Salivation.

Frequent necessity of expectoration. An indication of worms, and of mercurial poisoning.

Treatment.—For children: Ver. second dilution little and often. Unctions and compresses of C5 to the hypochondria.

For adults: S. alt. Ven. first dilution. Gargles of W. E.

Aphthæ.

Small white ulcerations on the lips, the mouth, or the digestive mucous membrane, attended with sense of illness, heat, pain in the mouth, fever, congestion of the glands on both sides of the jaw. The vesicles of the aphthous secretion ulcerate, and cicatrization is very slow.

Treatment.—Dil. S. or S. alt. C. Sometimes A2 alt. C5. Baths of C5, L. Gargles of C5, A2, S. (10 or 15 globules to the glass).

Inflammation of the Gums.

S., A., or C. in dilution. Gargles of C5 (15 globules to one glass of water), with W. E. alt. B. E. If there is congestion of blood to the head or to the gums, and bleeding of the latter, S. alt. A. Gargles of the same remedies and of B. E.

Palate: Polypus in the Palate.

Treatment.—C. in the second dilution. Same remedies in wine at meal-times. Gargles of C^4, C^5, A^2, W. E., R. E. Baths of C^5.

Tongue.

The tongue may be attacked in a secondary manner by all such inflammations as attack the mucous membranes of the throat. Ulceration and inflammation of the tongue.

Treatment.—C. in dilution or C^5, first dilution. C^5 in dilution, second dilution, may be tried. Gargles of the same remedies with W. E. or R. E. Baths of C^5. Unctions of C^5 to the hypochondria. Application of R. E. alt. Y. E. to the occiput and large and small hypoglossi.

Swelling of the Cheek.

Treatment.—S. Dil. second dilution. Application of R. E., and sometimes of R. E. alt. Y. E., to the sub-orbital region, the occiput, and under the ear.

Teeth (Diseases of the)

Toothache.—If it is a passing disorder resulting from cold or neuralgia, it can usually be removed by the application of W. E. to the temple and under the ear. R. E. and B. E. have often succeeded. If there is swelling, S. is necessary; if congestion, A. In obstinate cases, C.

Shrinking of the Gums.

Gargle of C^5 (20 globules to the glass of water). Gargle of W. E. or B. E.

Sub-Lingual Adhesions.

A disorder in which the tongue cannot move freely on account of adhesions to the floor of the mouth.

Treatment.—Dil. S. A. Gargle of A^2. Application of R. E. to the greater and lesser hypoglossi.

Dental Fistula.

Treatment.—Gargle of L. or of C^5 (20 globules to the glass). Unctions of F^2 to the hypochondria. Dil. S.

Difficult Dentition in Children.

Give to the nurse S. or A. Unctions of C^5 to the child's jaw.

Throat.

Sore Throat. Inflammation of the mucous membranes at the back of the mouth.

Treatment.—Simple sore throat requires A. and S. second dilution. If there is fever, remove it by F. second dilution, and dry globules of F. every hour until it disappears. If there is constipation, 20 globules of S. dry on the tongue on waking. Unctions of F^2 to the hypochondria. With or without fever, unctions of A^3 to the heart and on the throat. Application of R. E. alt. Y. E. to the large and small hypoglossi, of B. E. on the nape of the neck. If there is a cough add P.

Angina.

Inflammation of the mucous membranes lining the throat and the surrounding parts. There are several varieties: Guttural angina, angina tonsillaris, pharyngeal angina, and pseudo-membranous angina, with buff-coloured membrane.

Guttural Angina.

Pain and dryness in the throat, difficulty of swallowing;

the posterior wall of the pharynx looks red and slimy, secreting slowly a thready mucus which lines the tonsils and the arch of the palate. The uvula is swollen and elongated; there is an unpleasant taste in the mouth, offensive breath, loss of appetite, much thirst, diarrhœa or constipation, with fever of greater or less intensity. After three or four hours these symptoms abate.

In *treatment*, the constitution of the patient must be considered. If there is fever, it may be cut short at the outset by very frequent teaspoonful doses of F^1 every five or ten minutes, according to the case.

Dil. A. alt. S. second dilution. P. should be added if the bronchial tubes are affected—that is to say, if there is cough or expectoration. If the breath is fœtid or the case obstinate, give C. alone or S. alt. C.

Unctions of C^5 alt. A^2 to the whole of the throat. Unctions of A^3 to the heart. Gargles of R. E. or B.E. or Y. E. Application of R. E. alt. Y. E. to all the affected or central nerves. B. E. on the neck and head.

Angina Tonsillaris.

The symptoms resemble those of the preceding type. Inflammation attacks the tonsils, which become swollen, red, and hard. Suppuration and even gangrene may ensue.

Treatment.—Dil. A. alt. C. Then the same treatment as in the former variety.

Pharyngeal Angina.

Inflammation is seated in the upper or lower part of the pharyngeal mucous membrane. The surface is red, dry, covered with a greyish secretion. There is heat, smarting and dryness in the throat, as in guttural angina; but deglutition is easier, and there is less urging to swallow. To these symptoms there is added a cough, which provokes expulsion of the greyish mucus. If the cough changes its character and becomes hoarse and barking, there is reason to fear croup, especially in children.

Treatment.—Dil. A. or S. alt. C. Unctions of C^5 and A^3 to the entire throat. Gargle of R. E., B. E., or W. E., and C^5 (20 globules to a glass of water). Application to all the affected nerves of R. E. alt. Y. E. B. E. on the head and neck. Unctions of A^3 to the heart and of F^2 to the hypochondria.

Pseudo-Membranous Angina.

This angina is generally seated in the pharynx, the tonsils, the arches and roof of the palate. It is characterized by the formation of a false membrane, or skin, of a grey tint, which is apt to extend indefinitely over the adjacent parts.

Symptoms.—Convulsive cough, whistling respiration, sharp pain in the larynx, followed by loss of voice; then suffocation and often asphyxia. Small, weak, and frequent pulse, loss of power, putrid diarrhœa, or constipation and bilious vomiting. If the grey membrane invades the nasal fossæ bleeding ensues, and then a fœtid exudation of blood and matter.

Membranous formations may exist at any part within or behind the internal ear, around the nose and lips, or at the lower and aural orifices.

Treatment.—Dil. S. alt. A. second dilution: sometimes C. second dilution. One globule of C^5 every hour. Gargles of R. E., B. E., W. E., or C^5 (20 globules to the glass). Application of R. E. alt. Y. E. to the related nerves. Unctions of A^2 to the heart, and of F^2 to the hypochondria. Unctions and compresses of C^5 and A^2 to the entire throat.

Diphtheria.

A new remedy has been introduced, called Dom-fin, which is specific for diphtheria. For further directions for treatment, we refer the reader to the chapter on Laryngitis.

Amygdalitis.

See Angina Tonsillaris.

Cynanche (Quinsy).

See Angina.

FUNCTIONAL STOMACH DISORDERS.

Taste.

Loss of taste.

Treatment.—S. in dilution, first dilution. Application of R. E. to the pit of the stomach, and in compresses under the ears and on the nape of the neck.

Acidity.

A sign of bad digestion.

Treatment.—S. second dilution. Application of R. E. to the pit of the stomach.

Offensive Breath.

Treatment.—S. in dilution or C. first dilution. Gargles of R. E. or W. E. Application of R. E. alt. Y. E. to the solar plexus and pit of the stomach. Baths of C^5. Unctions to the pit of the stomach of C^5.

Appetite.

Loss of appetite should be treated by S., with baths of S. or L. or C^5. Persistent application of R. E. to the pit of the stomach.

Bulimy.

Almost insatiable hunger; so urgent that fainting arises if it is not satisfied. It is sometimes observed in hysteria, and more frequently in pregnancy.

Treatment.—Dil. S.; 5 globules of the same remedy, dry, three times a day. Baths of L.

Heartburn.

With or without pain.

Treatment.—C5 in dilution, or S. alt. A. Baths of C5. Unctions of C5. Compresses of W. E. or B. E. to the pit of the stomach.

Vomiting.

Treatment.—S. dil. second dilution. 10 globules of S., dry. The same treatment in pregnancy.

Periodical Vomiting.

Treatment.—F. dil. second dilution. Unctions of F2 to the hypochondria. Application of R. E. alt. Y. E. to the occiput, the sympathetic, and to the pit of the stomach. 10 globules dry of F. on waking. 1 globule of S. every hour.

Nausea.

Even during pregnancy.

Treatment.—C. in dilution, S., C5 in the first dilution: sipped frequently. Baths of C5. 1 globule of C2 every hour.

Sea-sickness.

Treatment.—S. in dilution, second dilution. 8 or 10 globules of S., dry, at each return of nausea.

Hæmatemesis.

Vomiting of blood. This affection arises from an effusion of blood in the interior of the stomach, which rejects it by the œsophagus and by the mouth. This hæmorrhage is one of the less frequent, and rarely occurs except in middle life, between the thirtieth and fiftieth year, among individuals of a nervous temperament, lean constitution, melancholic disposition, and who lead a sedentary life. Excess of food, an emetic injudiciously taken, painful emotion, irregular menstruation, or the suppression of some other hæmorrhage, are sometimes the occasional causes of hæmatemesis. This hæmorrhage is much more often symptomatic than idiopathic.

The vomiting of blood is sometimes preceded by coldness in the extremities, heat and heaviness at the epigastrium, pallor of the face, oppression, fainting, buzzing in the ears, giddiness, loss of strength, syncopy, sweetish taste in the mouth.

The general phenomena are the same as those accompanying other hæmorrhages.

Sometimes there is only one vomiting of blood; more often they occur after intervals of several hours, or several days. The duration of this condition is difficult to determine, and can only be known approximately, according to the time that the expulsion of blood lasts, either above or below.

After this hæmorrhage, those who survive have a wan, pale face, œdema in the legs, and slow digestion. With some cases the disorder returns periodically.

Treatment.—During hæmorrhage, A^2 second dilution, a teaspoonful to be taken every five minutes. Gargles of B. E. Enemata of S. Application of R. E. by cupping to the soles of the feet. To prevent hæmorrhage: A. alt. C. in ordinary doses. To guard against the effects of hæmorrhage: Baths, with 100 globules of A^1. Friction in the dorsal region of R. E.

SOBBING, OR HICCOUGH.

Nervous contraction of the diaphragm, with flatulence. This is sometimes destroyed by a simple application of R. E. to the occiput and to the pit of the stomach. If obstinate, use S. dil. or C^5 second dilution.

Several globules of S^1, taken dry, generally stop it.

SPASMS, OR CRAMP OF THE STOMACH.

If they are accidental they ordinarily yield to 10 globules of S. dry, and R. E. to the pit of the stomach.

GASTRALGIA.

Disorder characterized by sharp, shooting, cutting, tearing, or burning pain, or by a feeling of pressure, swelling, or tympanitis. This pain spreads to the back as far as the shoulders, is often accompanied by constipation, distension, eructations, nausea, sometimes anxiety, suffocation, faintness, or even delirium, and a flow of liquid or glairy matters into the mouth. Appetite good, excepting in chronic cases.

Treatment.—Simple stomach pains are easily cured by S. in dilution, second dilution. The same remedy in wine at meal-time. 1 globule of S., dry, every hour, or 20 globules, dry, of S^5 on waking in the morning. Baths of C^5, of S^5 or W. E. Unctions of F^2 to the hypochondria, and of C^5 to the stomach. Application of R. E. alt. Y. E. to the sympathetic nerve and the epigastrium. If an obstinate case, C. alt. Ver. and use of B. E. Unctions of F^2 to the hypochondria. Application of R. E. to the pit of the stomach.

GASTRALGIA.

Accompanied by periodical vomitings, pain or cramp;—may be survivals of old syphilis.

Treatment.—F. in dilution alt. Ven. The same remedies at meal-time (from 5 to 10 globules). Baths of C^5, S^5 alt. Ven. Unctions of F^2 to the hypochondria. Application of R. E. alt. Y. E. to the sympathetic nerve and solar plexus.

DISTENSION OR DILATATION OF THE STOMACH.

Treatment.—S. in dilution alt. C^5. The same remedies at meal-time. Baths of C^5 or W. E. Unctions of C^5 on the stomach, and of F^2 to the hypochondria. Application of R. E. alt. Y. E. to the sympathetic nerve and solar plexus, or W. E. to the pit of the stomach.

Dyspepsia: Indigestion.

Always associated with a lymphatic type of constitution. Food lies heavy on the stomach; sense of illness; pain, yawning, frequent eructation or belching, acid rising, nausea, distension, constipation or diarrhœa, or alternation of each; heaviness of the head, muddled; melancholy disposition; and irritability, or depression of spirits.

Treatment.—Slow or arrested digestion may be restored by dry globules of S., and application of R. E. to the pit of the stomach. 10 or 20 globules of S. dry on the tongue prevent indigestion when only just beginning. If this is not successful, take S. or S^5 in the first dilution, or 1 globule of S. dry every half-hour. Application of R. E. to the pit of the stomach. Unctions of F^2 to the hypochondria.

Bilious Dyspepsia.

If dyspepsia arises from bilious conditions, the disorder is aggravated by the action of S., and disappears by the use of F^1 in dil. and unctions of F^2 to the hypochondria. Apply R. E. to the pit of the stomach.

Digestion.

Special Characteristics of Disorders of the Digestive System.—Every one knows that digestion means the introduction of solids or liquids into special cavities; which substances are changed in these cavities, and are then absorbed and distributed to the different tissues, to which they supply nutrition. This great physiological function is allotted to many different organs: accordingly the symptoms which characterize disorders of the digestive system arise from changes produced in one or more of these organs, which constitute the different portions of a complex mechanism. The whole work of digestion can only be perfectly done when all the component parts of this machine work in a regular and harmonious way.

Thus *Œsophagitis*, which is simply inflammation of the first portion of the intestinal conduit—that which, being continuous with the mouth and throat, extends from the pharynx to the cardiac orifice of the stomach—prevents deglutition, or at any rate causes acute pain and difficulty in an act which ought to be passive and spontaneous.

Gastritis causes either vomiting, or pain and serious illness. *Enteritis* causes diarrhœa or constipation. In disorders of the liver, the bile, instead of flowing into the duodenum, and aiding digestion, may be absorbed, and give rise to jaundice, or icterus, so easily recognized by the yellow colour of the skin and the conjunctiva of the eye, and the deep colour of the urine.

These conditions are easily met by the use of S^1, unctions of F^2, and applications of R. E. alt. Y. E. Also S^1 and A^1 may be alternated.

Three kinds of obstruction may resist the descent of the food from the mouth to the stomach.

1. *Œsophagitis*, or inflammation of the gullet.
2. Nervous or spasmodic contraction.
3. Organic contraction of the mucous membrane of the œsophagus, the membrane being gathered into folds like rings.

The first two are treated by S^1, sometimes alternated with A^2. But the third requires the internal use of C^1 in order to cure the mucous thickening which is the essential obstruction to digestion.

To cure *Gastritis*, gastric irritation, and even acute gastritis, we must employ S^1 and applications of R. E. alt. Y. E.

Non-bilious dyspepsia, gastritis, indeed all disorders of this kind, which are equally baffling to doctors and patient, are cured by S^1 and applications of R. E. Every one is familiar with the symptoms of these maladies, and description for the purposes of this work is needless.

But there is an obstinate disorder which has hitherto

resisted all treatment—I mean gastralgia, or gastric cramp or spasm; which, when it is obstinate, acts so strongly on the mental and moral condition of the patient as almost invariably to bring on hypochondriasis. It assumes a thousand different forms, as it may arise from as many different causes. Nevertheless the electro-homœopathic specifics are always able to cope with this disease, which has resisted the treatment of the most distinguished practitioners. How many unhappy persons, tormented by the most horrible sufferings, exhausted and almost at death's door, have sought relief from these specifics, and have been not only relieved but cured!

To the hygienic and dietetic treatment which are imperative in the management of these disorders, a dual electro-homœopathic treatment is added; on the one hand the neuralgic pains must be removed, on the other hand the disease itself must be eradicated. If it is chronic its periodicity must be destroyed, and the accidental causes must be encountered.

For this purpose we must resort to S. in the smallest doses (that is, the second or third dilutions) during the paroxysm; and to unctions of F^2 to the hypochondria, and application of R. E.; subsequently to S. in the first dilution, and this must be continued for some time if the cure is to be radical. It is scarcely possible to be too assiduous in the treatment of these neuralgic types of gastric disorder, which are so liable to relapse.

The same treatment is also efficacious in a more transient affection, which may, however, assume distressing intensity,—that is, hiccough or spasm of the diaphragm. The diaphragm, being suddenly contracted, gives a sharp shock to the thoracic and abdominal cavities, accompanied by a peculiar dull sound and a sudden contraction of the glottis, with impeded respiration. As we have said, in the great majority of cases hiccough is a trifling and passing disorder which ceases of itself in a few minutes. But frequently it appears in some abdominal disorders, peritonitis for example, and may then indicate the approach of a fatal termination.

As it does not form part of our plan to describe all varieties of abdominal disease, and we refer only incidentally to such an ordinary symptom, we need only advise—for hiccough resulting from simple contraction of the diaphragm, occurring mostly when the stomach is quite full, and especially when the patient has been eating heavy food fast and without drinking—the treatment just indicated, with application of R. E. to the pit of the stomach. If, on the contrary, it is symptomatic of some abdominal disease, on the principle that all nervous abdominal disorders start from the phrenic or diaphragmatic centre, adjoining the pillars of the diaphragm, we must employ F., and often even C., which is of the highest efficacy in these numerous neuroses in all their various disguises.

At present we desire especially to consider disorders of digestion, and the best means of preventing or retarding them. We find by experience that all the symptoms of various forms of dyspepsia are met by these remedies. Bilious dyspepsia, however, requires the internal and external use of F.

S. is always able to arrest the rising of food, purify the mouth when it is bitter or slimy, and to encounter all disorders of this class. It may even remove the discomfort often caused by the pressure of the clothes on the epigastrium at the commencement of digestion.

We must use A. alternately with S. against chronic and inveterate cases of gastritis, caused by irritation of the nerves distributed over the mucous membrane of the stomach, always attended by insatiable thirst, by redness of the margin and tip of the tongue, with smarting heat on the palm of the hand after food. Often C. alt. A. is better.

In all cases of indigestion it is necessary to use S. This is emphatically the remedy; it disperses these functional disorders and arrests the development of still graver diseases. Certain other diseases, such as intense thirst, vomiting, &c., arising from a nervous cause, if they do not entirely yield to S., are certainly subdued by the use of C., and sometimes by A. alt. F.

C. alt. A. are equally efficacious in arresting vomiting of blood, arising from cancer of the pylorus. The constant use of these remedies in dilution or unctions, assisted by the application of the electricities, have always relieved and often cured a crowd of unhappy sufferers afflicted with diseases of this kind; among others, the Countess Chiassi, of Rome, who was cured of cancer of the pylorus. (See the *Cancer* section.)

Bilious vomiting, being an indication of great disorder of the liver, requires the use of the Febrifugos, which meet both the causes and effects of this disease.

Among the varieties of vomiting we must refer to a serious and dangerous disorder, which may result from strangulated hernia, or intus-susception of the intestines—that is, ileus, or stercoraceous vomiting. To meet this grave disorder, S. alt. C. in dilution must be used; sometimes a dilution of A. and enemata of C^5. Unctions of C^5 on the abdomen must be added, and W. E. applied to the skull and the great sympathetic.

Affections of the liver, acute or chronic hepatitis, hepatalgia, with pains in the right shoulder-blade which indicate the presence of liver disorder, icterus, congestion of the liver, hypochondriasis, bilious melancholy, in subjects characterized by a bilious temperament, form a group of disorders in which the curative power of F. and F^a are conspicuous.

Disorders of the spleen, acute or chronic splenitis, splenalgia, chronic congestion of this organ resulting from intermittent fever, and, in a word, all diseases of the spleen or liver, require the use of these same specifics in dilution, and externally as compresses on the hypochondrium.

Another disease requires much more careful observation

in making a diagnosis, namely, pancreatitis or inflammation of the pancreas. It is known that this gland, which has a great anatomical resemblance to the salivary glands, is intended to secrete a fluid by which fatty matters may be dissolved and converted into chyle.

Diseases of this organ, especially those of inflammatory type, which are always slow, announce themselves by symptoms which may be detected by touch, in a limited space situated between the lesser lobe of the liver and the small curve of the stomach. But a more unequivocal indication of this disorder is the absolute impossibility of digesting fatty substances, and consequently an unconquerable aversion to all food of this kind. There is also another symptom which depends upon the pathological and physiological sympathy which connects these two organs with a similar structure; and that is abundant salivation and an excessively perverted condition of the salivary secretion, which is required for primary digestion. For all these affections we must use F. and the application of R.E. The results are positive, and are attested by a thousand instances.

There is one point on which we must insist. We all know the intimate dependence of the state of the brain and that of the digestive apparatus. But it is not sufficiently considered what great influence gastritis, hepatitis, and creeping splenitis exercise on the undisturbed action of the mental and intellectual faculties. If we leave insanity and monomania, of various types, out of consideration, which proceed from causes directly connected with the cerebral nervous system, we may safely assert that the original seat of nearly all nervous diseases is either the stomach, the liver, or the spleen. If we watch carefully the state of the unfortunate victims of these disorders, we shall be able to detect in all of them some digestive disorder. If we examine the epigastric region, we generally find that the least pressure causes severe pain. The skin is almost always cold, and this is a symptom which infallibly indicates deep-seated disease in the ganglionic abdominal system and the alimentary tract. The tongue is always rather dry, and coated with bilious deposit, looking as if the patient had been chewing rhubarb. These pathological observations are equally confirmed by the phenomena of hypochondriasis—an exaggerated and morbid self-consciousness in regard to health—which is nothing more than a species of monomania, and the seat of it is undoubtedly the stomach. In certain temperaments of a markedly hepatic type, the venous system exerts a material dynamic action which cannot be ignored. In consequence of a change in the functions of the liver, caused by violent pain, especially when the manifestation of it is violently suppressed, a hepatic, venous congestion arises, of slow type, by which the liver is prevented from eliminating from the organism the hydro-carbons which, when retained, always give rise to serious illness. The biliary secretion is chemically changed; it becomes acrid, black, thicker than ordinary; it cannot pass freely into the duodenum, and ceases to contribute its important functional aid in the work of digestion.

As soon as the bile is arrested for a certain time in any one portion of the liver, it is absorbed, and, being mixed with the circulation, affects the nervous system and excites its sensibilities. Thus an excess of bile in the blood may occasion those quick bursts of anger which are so characteristic of the hepatic temperament, whether original, or induced by disease of the organ. If these phenomena are only transient, if the hepatic disorder comes to an end, these disorders of the nervous system also subside and tranquillity is restored. But if, on the contrary, this abnormal condition of the liver, and indirectly also of the spleen and of the abdominal venous circulation, is prolonged, it is plain that an influence so marked must act continuously on the cerebral nervous system, and leave traces on the finest mental qualities, bringing inevitably more or less confirmed insanity or monomania. The practitioner who is in search of originating causes will always in such cases examine the liver, and find its smaller lobe congested; there is tumefaction of the abdomen, &c. Moreover, it will not be difficult to establish the existence of gas lodged in the intestines, arising from the decomposition of bile charged with an excess of carbonaceous principles. The moral state of the patient is always depressed and gloomy. One of the characteristic symptoms of such disorders is a blackish patch which appears at the root of the tongue, of a triangular form, the point always directed outwards; and this patch becomes more or less developed according as the disease takes greater or diminishing proportions.

This purely pathological digression which we have ventured to introduce is simply designed to accentuate the enormous influence which the electro-homœopathic specifics are able to exert on a large number of psychic or moral affections which are dependent on some abnormal state of the liver or the spleen. In these cases we cannot too assiduously push the action of F. taken internally, and F^2 used in compresses to the hypochondria. A. and S. in small doses, with unctions of C. along the dorsal spine, and application of R. E. and Y. E., are also necessary. We are fortunately in a position to affirm that the efficacy of the electro-homœopathic remedies has been so repeatedly demonstrated that doubt on this point is impossible.

Inflammations of the small and large intestines, or colic, form a group which varies infinitely in character and gradation: the causes and symptoms are multiform. Nevertheless, if taken in time, these diseases are easily cured by Electro-Homœopathy. The best specific for diseases of the intestines is C., with a minute dose of A. internally. Sometimes it will be well to use unctions of C^5 or of F^2 to the hypochondria, and baths of L., with application of R. E. Constipation, as well as diarrhœa and dysentery, are nothing else than disturbances of the regular action of the digestive apparatus induced by various causes. Epidemic or autumnal diarrhœa, mucous diarrhœa, are maladies which require prompt and assiduous attention, because they may lead to still graver disorders and a tendency to ulceration. The treatment begins with S., alt. in certain cases with A. But if amelioration is not established we must have recourse to C^5 alt. A. internally, to unctions of F^2 to the hypochondria, with application of R. E. and Y. E. alternately. After some time, when the primary improvement sets in, we may discontinue external treatment, and limit ourselves to internal; that is to say, to C. administered in larger doses, in order to avoid the ulcerative destruction which is the predominant characteristic of these infirmities; and thus always tends to the complete destruction of the organism.

One of the disorders which it is well to note is inflammation of the peritonæum, the great serous membrane which covers the intestines. As soon as peritonitis has been diagnosed—and the diagnosis is easy—we must immediately have recourse to energetic treatment by A. alt. with C. And if the patient has a sanguine temperament, A. must be added. Also the patient should take 8 or 10 globules of F. every morning on waking. External treatment must be superadded in the form of unctions of C^5 on the abdomen, and of F^2 on the hypochondria; application of W. E. and even baths of C^5 and A^2.

There are numerous forms of intestinal neuralgia; enteralgia, or spasm of the rectum; different forms of gastric colic; intestinal or nervous colic, or spasmodic, inflammatory; saturnine or lead colic; bilious colic, caused by some disappointment, or moral and emotional suffering; flatulent colic; disorders of the cæcum: these are disorders which trouble the exercise of the gastro-intestinal viscera. All these disorders yield to the regular use of S. alt. C. in the first, second, or third dilution, according to the intensity of the disease. This is the internal treatment. Externally we must use R. E. alt. Y. E. Often also we must resort to C^5.

In these disorders we cannot dispense with the use of Ver.; some globules at bedtime. This specific always produces excellent results.

Nervous Gastritis.

Treatment.—F. in dilution. Unctions of F² to the hypochondria. Application of W. E. to the sympathetic nerve and solar plexus. Baths of C5, and, three times a day, 3 drops of W. E. on a piece of sugar.

ABDOMINAL DISEASES.

The Abdomen

Is bounded above by the diaphragm, below by the pelvis, behind by the lumbar vertebræ, laterally and in front by many large and flat muscles, the fibres of which cross in different directions. Its form is oblong, convex anteriorly and still more inferiorly, concave behind and laterally. Its form and volume are liable to an indefinite number of variations, according to circumstances.

The posterior wall is divided into two regions only, the superior or lumbar, otherwise called the loins, and the inferior or sacral region. The lateral walls of the abdomen have three divisions on each side; the upper or hypochondrium; the middle or the lumbar lateral region; and the lower or iliac, called also the iliac fossæ. The upper wall is formed by a sort of roof which represents the diaphragm. The lower part includes two regions; the anterior or genital, and the posterior, or rectal and anal. These two regions are separated in both sexes by a space called the perinæum.

The diseases of the abdomen are very numerous, and include all those that affect the liver, the mesentery, the intestines, the ovaries, the urino-generative system. In all intestinal disorders, after a short trial of S. use A., as there may be some orgasm of the blood; or C., the great remedy for intestinal disorder.

General Treatment.—S. or A. in dilution, first dilution. 1 globule of S. every half-hour, or 10 at a time, dry. Unctions of C^5 to the pit of the stomach. Sometimes compresses of F^2 also to the pit of the stomach. C^5 in dilution. Baths of C^5. Application of R. E. alt. Y. E. to the pit of the stomach, sympathetic, loins, and to the lower part of the dorsal spine on both sides. Unctions of C^5 on the stomach, and compresses of W. E. on the same part.

Weakness of the Intestines.

Treatment.—S. in dilution, first dilution. 1 globule of C^5 or S. every half-hour. Baths of C^5. Compresses of W. E. Application of R. E. alt. Y. E. to the sympathetic, solar plexus, and down each side of the dorsal spine.

Periodical Inflammation of the Intestines.

Treatment.—F. in dilution alt. C^5 (second dilution). 1 globule of C^5 every half-hour. In other respects treat as for intestinal weakness; but with more use of unctions of F^2 to the hypochondria.

Ascites; or Abdominal Dropsy.

Dropsy of the abdomen means an accumulation of serum or serous fluid in the cavity of the peritonœum. If there is any disorder in the circulation this kind of dropsy may arise from the state of the heart.

Treatment.—Dilution of A. or A. alt. S. in small doses, the second dilution. No electricity, unless it be blue. Application of A^2 over the heart.

The liver may be the origin of the dropsy, and then we must give F. in dil. or F. alt. S., second dilution, and the same remedies at meals. Unction of F^2 to the hypochondria.

Dropsy may proceed from the mesenteric gland. In this

case we must give C. dil. or C. alt. S., second dilution; and the same remedies at meals. Unction of F^2 or C^5 to the hypochondria.

Enteritis.

Inflammation of the bowels. At the commencement there is but little fever; the abdomen is swollen and tender or painful; appetite lost or diminished. The patient suffers from dull, colicky pain, or acute and lancinating pains around the umbilicus; then these colics extend all over the stomach; diarrhœa of yellow substances mixed with mucous; the anus is burning and tender. If the colic subsides, rumbling of wind remains, and if this continues headache follows, fainting, nausea, vomiting. If the inflammation attacks the mucous membrane of the stomach as well as that of the intestines, the case is one of gastro-enteritis.

Treatment.—Dil. S. or S. alt C.; the same remedies at meals. 1 globule of C^5 every hour. Baths of C^5 or L. Compresses of B. E. over the abdomen. Application of R. E. alt. Y. E. to the solar plexus, to the pit of the stomach, to the sympathetic at the stomach, occiput, and grand sympathetic centre. Unction of C^5 over the whole abdomen.

Mesenteritis.

Inflammation or tubercular disease of the mesenteric glands; called also *tabes mesenterica*, or *marasmus*. Is only developed in infants or young children from five to ten years old.

Symptoms.—Pallor of the face, feebleness, diarrhœa alternating with constipation; round and hard swelling in the region of the navel; sometimes cough and night sweats; tongue normal; appetite preserved notwithstanding emaciation, wasting of the limbs, low spirits, and frequent crying; then, at last, hectic fever, rapid prostration, and death.

Treatment.—Dil. C., second dilution. 1 globule of C^5,

dry, every hour; baths of C^5; unctions of L.; and compresses of B. E. over the abdomen. Application of B. E. to the sympathetic; unctions of F^2 to the hypochondria.

Intestinal Phthisis.

Is recognized by bad digestion, and especially by pain and tension of the abdomen, and evacuation of pus mixed with blood. This disease is attended by hectic fever.

Treatment.—Dil. of S. or L.; or, in obstinate cases, S. alt. C. 1 globule of C^5 dry every hour.

Ditto for Sanguine Temperaments.—A. alt. S. Baths of C^5, alternating with S^5 or A^2. Unctions or compresses of C^5 over the abdomen, also of B. E. Application of B. E. to the sympathetic.

Peritonitis.

Inflammation of the lining membrane of the abdomen and bowels. It may be either acute or chronic.

Symptoms.—Severe, sharp, lancinating pains, increased by the least pressure on the abdomen. Constipation; vomiting; breathing, short, rapid, and oppressed; frequent pulse; great change of expression in the face; difficult digestion; effusion of serous fluid. Peritonitis may be complicated by ataxic symptoms, such as mild or furious delirium; adynamic symptoms, such as prostration of the vital forces, tongue dry, brown, or black; somnolence; involuntary evacuation and urination; bilious symptoms, jaundiced or sallow tint, bloated appearance, bitter taste, bilious vomiting.

Treatment.—10 globules of F^1 dry in the morning. Dil. S. alt. S. second dilution; 1 globule of C^5 every hour. For angioitic persons, A. alt. S. or A. alt. L. Baths of C^5, or S^5, or A^3. Unctions and compresses of C^5 or F^2 on the abdomen and hypochondria. Application of B. E. to the sympathetic; 5 drops of the same on the scalp.

MISERERE OR ILEUS.

A disease characterized by pain deep in the abdomen, vomiting of the contents of the stomach and intestines, and obstinate constipation.

Nervous temperaments, youth, a strong moral impression, some irregularity in diet, have been indicated as the most ordinary causes. Symptomatic ileus is generally produced by closure of the intestinal canal, by internal or external strangulation. The principal symptoms are a violent pain, sometimes intolerable, in the abdomen, with a kind of movement of the intestines in this cavity, contraction, and hardness of the abdominal walls, gaseous eructations, then vomiting of the contents of the stomach, then of the small intestine, and still later of the large intestine. Evidently, as the disease advances, the substances successively rejected are each time from a more distant part of the intestinal canal, and end in presenting the aspect and odour of stercoraceous matter. In some cases even, according to some authorities, liquids injected into the rectum, or suppositories placed in the bowel, have been ejected through the mouth. Constipation is persistent throughout the course of the disease, in some cases reaching such a point that even wind cannot be discharged. To these local symptoms are added sudden and marked alteration of the features, discolouration of the face, bending forwards of the body, anxiety, discouragement, weak voice, dyspnœa, fainting, convulsive movements, stercoraceous fœtor of the breath, small and irregular pulse, coldness of the extremities, cold perspiration, increasing prostration of strength.

Ileus often has exacerbations; sometimes the intensity of the symptoms takes a fairly regular progress. It increases rapidly, and in a few days it ends in death. Hiccough, delirium, unsuccessful efforts to vomit, aphonia, imperceptibility of the pulse, precede and announce death.

In some cases, after an apparent cure, the symptoms return with the same intensity and even greater danger.

Treatment.—5 globules of S. dry on the tongue every hour. S. or C. in dilution, second or third dilution, sipped frequently. Compresses of F^2 to the hypochondria. Application of R. E. to the sacrum, perinæum, and sympathetic. Every hour an enema of 8 ounces of water medicated with 15 globules of C^5. Compresses and unctions of C^5 over the abdomen

LIVER AND SPLEEN DISORDERS.

These are two viscera of primary rank. Disorder of the liver is usually attended by a yellow tint of the skin and of the whites of the eyes ; thick, yellow or reddish urine ; grey, clayey evacuations, constipation, pain in the right side or at the pit of the stomach, extending to the dorsal spine and up to the right shoulder and the neck, with heaviness on the right side, and often bilious vomitings and bitter taste in the mouth, especially in the morning.

Nearly all disorders of the liver and spleen affect the stomach and intestines, especially when they are of an inflammatory character and cause ordinary gastralgia, which, instead of being relieved by S., like simple gastralgia, increase under its influence and resist it. It is by this indication that we recognize the fact that the disorder originates in the liver.

The heart also sympathizes with disorders of the liver, and in addition to the symptoms mentioned there also appears giddiness and palpitation, when F. alt. A^2, second dilution, must be used, and unctions added of A^2 on the heart, and of F^2 on the hypochondria. 3 drops of W. E. on sugar three times a day is useful as a protection against liver attacks.

Congestion of the Liver with Dropsy.

Treatment.—F. in dilution alt. C., second dilution. 1 globule of F. every hour. Baths of A. alt. F^2. Unctions of

F² on the hypochondria. Unctions of A3 on the heart. Applications of R. E. alt. Y. E. to the solar plexus and sympathetic nerve. 5 globules C5 dry on waking.

Tumour on the Liver.

Treatment.—F. in dilution alt. C5. Baths of C5 alt. F². Unctions of F² to the hypochondria. Applications of R. E. alt. Y. E. to the grand sympathetic, solar plexus, and the pit of the stomach.

Icterus, Jaundice.

Yellow discolouration of the skin, consequent on the passage of the bile into the blood, with thick yellow, or red and scanty urine, evacuations of a grey ash or silvery colour.

Treatment.—F¹ in dilution, second dilution. Baths of C5. Unctions of F² to the hypochondria. Applications of R. E. alt. Y. E. to the occiput and sympathetic, or B. E. 3 drops of W. E. on a piece of sugar three times a day.

Gastro-hepatitis.

Acute or chronic inflammation of the liver and stomach, with heavy pains in the right side; enlarged liver, difficult respiration, painful digestion, eructations, constipation or diarrhœa, sometimes evacuations mixed with blood; pale or yellow skin, emaciation, with abdominal inflation.

Treatment.—10 globules of F. dry on waking. F. in dilution alt. A., alt. L., second dilution.. Three times a day 3 drops of W. E. on a piece of sugar. Unctions of F² to the hypochondria. Unctions of A3 to the heart, and C5 down the back. Applications of R. E. alt. Y. E. to the grand sympathetic, solar plexus, and pit of the stomach.

Biliary Calculi.

Produce excessively severe colic, termed hepatic colic. These calculi are expelled with the stools.

Treatment.—Dil. S^2 alt. F. Same remedies at meals. Baths of S. alt. F^2. Unctions of F^2 to the hypochondria. 10 globules of F. on waking, dry, on the tongue.

Hepatitis.

Local symptoms: pain in the region of the liver, a feeling of heaviness, a tumour of large or small dimensions, flattened, smooth, hard, terminated below by a narrow angular ridge or border parallel to that of the chest; disordered secretion of bile, which is suspended or changed. The gastric digestion is slow, painful, and imperfect; the evacuations are scanty and seldom; fæcal matter is changed in consistency or colour, being often grey or ash-coloured, very hard or very soft. The complexion is nearly always yellowish; the bulk and vigour of the body diminish slowly; as a rule it is only after a long time that the pulse is accelerated, and a sort of hectic fever is established, with nocturnal perspirations. Some patients succumb by falling into a dropsical state, others by extreme wasting and exhaustion.

Treatment.—The treatment is quite simple, but once begun, must not be discontinued until the cure is complete; relapse is fatal to the patient. Internally, A. alt. F., second or third dilution. Externally, three times a day, F^2 in compresses on the hypochondria. If there is no very great improvement, C^1, and its varieties must be resorted to externally and internally. Unctions or compresses of C^5 or F^2 on the hypochondria. Applications of R. E. alt. Y. E. on the sympathetic nerve, to the pit of the stomach, occiput, and solar plexus.

Hypochondriasis.

This disease has been so named because it has been supposed that its origin or seat is in these regions. It is characterized by an extreme susceptibility of the nervous system, morose disposition, often accompanied by flatulence and different disorders of the digestive organs.

Treatment.—S. in dilution alt. F., third dilution. Application of R. E. to the grand sympathetic, solar plexus, occiput, and pit of the stomach. Unction of F^2 to the hypochondria.

Spleen.

Diseases of the spleen, like tænia, produce very strange phenomena. They simulate all sorts of grave diseases. The enlargement of its volume, and the disturbance thus caused by pressure on adjacent viscera, are the causes of these symptoms.

In splenitis or acute inflammation of the spleen, the following are the symptoms: General feebleness, pain in the left hypochondrium extending to the shoulder, painful swelling about the ribs, loss of appetite, thirst, nausea or vomiting, sometimes fever with agitation, delirium, suffocation, &c.

Treatment.—Dil. F., second dilution. The same remedy dry (4 globules at each meal), 1 globule of C^5 every hour. Three times a day, 3 drops of W. E. on a lump of sugar. Baths of C^5 or W. E. (a tablespoonful to the bath). Unctions of F^2 to the hypochondria. Application of R. E. alt. Y. E. to the sympathetic, solar plexus, and occiput.

Pancreatitis.

Inflammation of the pancreas sometimes shows itself in the course of bad fevers, typhoid or puerperal, or from the effects of phlebitis (inflammation of the veins) or of mercury.

The principal symptoms are: Fixed pain at the epigastrium, extending under the right hypochondrium, accompanied with heat at the same point, with intestinal flux of colourless thin fluid like saliva, tightness of the abdomen, swelling of the pancreatic region, fever, loss of appetite, and sometimes vomiting or jaundice. These are the indications of acute disease of the pancreas.

Chronic inflammation of the pancreas, which has been less observed than acute, is habitually characterized by constant salivation; watery, thin eructations, of a yellowish colour; constipation, or diarrhœa of a fluid similar to that which is thrown out by the mouth; lastly, want of appetite, pyrosis, and very marked gastralgia, or stomach neuralgia.

Treatment.—Dil. S. alt. F. Baths of C^5. Unctions of F^2 to the hypochondria. Application of R. E. alt. Y. E. to the sympathetic.

Hernia, or Rupture.

Abnormal tumour formed by any viscus which escapes from its proper cavity or confining walls, and appears on the surface.

Treatment.—S. in dilution alt. A., first or second dilution. Application by compresses of R. E. or W. E. or B. E. on the hernia and solar plexus. Baths. Unctions and compresses of C^5 and S^5.

Colics.

Sharp pains extending through the whole of the abdomen, but especially severe about the navel. Altered face, hands and feet cold, abundant perspiration, discharge of flatulence, which gives relief.

The attack is often sudden; the expression of the face immediately changes; the patient is in a singular state of depression and agitation.

Treatment.—Dil. S. in small and repeated doses; 1 globule of S. every half-hour. Application of R. E. alt. Y. E. to the pit of the stomach. Unctions of C^5 over the abdomen. In obstinate cases C^5 in dilution.

Hepatic Colic.

Dil. F. alt. A., second dilution. Unctions of F^2 to the hypochondria and of C^5 to the abdomen. Three times a day take 4 drops of W. E. on a piece of sugar. Baths of S. L. alt. F^2. Application of W. E.

ENTERALGIA, OR NERVOUS COLIC.

The symptoms are, severe pain all over the abdomen, especially severe at the navel; changed appearance; cold hands and feet; abundant sweats; belching or rumbling of wind, and much escape of wind by eructation or evacuation.

Treatment.—S^2 to be taken in dil. frequently; 1 globule of S^2 dry, every hour. Baths of C^5. Application of B. E. to the sympathetic, and unctions of C^5 to the abdomen.

CONSTIPATION

Proceeds either from excitement of the blood, or the intestines, or the womb.

Treatment.—For lymphatics, dil. S. and 10 globules of the same remedy dry, night and morning.

For angioitics, the same treatment with A.

In some circumstances constipation has been met by 3 globules of Ver. in a large glassful of water, taken in three or four draughts.

MELÆNA.

Vomiting of black blood, flow of black blood from the digestive apparatus and escaping from the mouth or the bowel.

(*See* Vomitings.)

DIARRHŒA.

A disease characterized by frequent alvine evacuations; it arises from inflammation or irritation of the mucous membrane of the intestines.

Treatment.—If there is no blood in the stools: dil. S.; also 10 or 20 globules of S. dry. Baths of S^5 or C^5. Application of R. E. alt Y. E. to the sympathetic, solar plexus, and pit of the stomach. Scrofoloso giappone must always be resorted to if diarrhœa is obstinate.

If there is blood in the stools: dil. A. alt. S.; 10 globules dry, of A^2. Baths of A^3 alt. C^5. Unctions of C^5 to the abdomen, of A^3 to the heart, and of F^2 to the hypochondria.

Dysentery.

Inflammation of the mucous membrane of the large intestine, especially the rectum, characterized by pain in the abdomen, and evacuation of mucus, which is generally bloody. All parts of the intestinal canal may be affected in dysentery, but the rectum is almost always more affected than the rest of the intestines, and sometimes it alone is involved.

Dysentery occurs especially in summer and autumn, when the atmosphere is humid, and the changes of temperature are rapid and extreme. It is more common in low and marshy districts, with a south or west aspect; also in prisons, in camps, and among persons suffering from privation and want. Dysentery is generally considered contagious.

Among the general symptoms which are attendant upon dysentery, we may remark especially the depressed expression of the face, pallor, languor, and extreme weakness, headache, sleeplessness, thirst, difficult digestion, accelerated pulse, transient shivering.

Treatment.—Dil. A. alt. C., 1 globule of C^5 every hour. Unctions to the hypochondria of F^2 and of C^5 to the abdomen. Application of R. E. alt. Y. E. to the grand sympathetic, solar plexus, the occiput, and pit of the stomach.

Cholera

Is a well marked disease of quite peculiar type, assuming the most formidable aspects. It seems to have originated on the banks of the Ganges, and then visited at different times nearly all the countries of Europe and the world, everywhere bringing terror, desolation, and death. This is Asiatic Cholera.

Although this fearful scourge attacks at one stroke the entire organism, it is not to be denied that the intestinal canal is the part where it is most developed, where its attack is most felt, and the resulting disorder the most severe. And yet the imminent danger attendant upon this disease, and the nature of the disease itself, have nothing in common with the ordinary ailments of the intestinal canal. The true cause of cholera is nothing less than a subtle poison pervading the air, a poison at once contagious and epidemic, which eludes the impressions of our senses and insinuates itself into the organism through respiration, or by the pores of the skin, and perhaps also by the gastro-enteric apparatus.

The dreadful symptoms of this disease, its innumerable victims, even the striking peculiarities of its invasion and development, have unfortunately made its characteristics familiar to multitudes. Moreover, its epidemic character, and all the alarming circumstances which attend it, do not leave a shadow of doubt upon its diagnosis when it is really present. Without entering upon any physiological or pathological considerations—for this would involve many long and curious digressions, which however are not without important bearings upon practice—without also dilating on the history of this disease, which would be essential if our object were to give complete directions for treatment, we shall limit ourselves to a concise and accurate description of the different stages which it may pass through.

The course of the disease may be divided into three periods: the period of invasion, the algide period, and the period of reaction.

1. *Prodomata, or Invasion.*—Most usually the invasion stage of Asiatic cholera is preceded by prodomata or pre-

monitory symptoms sufficient to indicate the nature of the approaching attack. These symptoms are especially significant if there is an epidemic already existing. Very commonly the approach of the disease is marked by gastric disturbance, a sort of gastric catarrh lasting several days. In a multitude of cases the premonitory symptoms are as follows: Indescribable *malaise* and rapid loss of strength, weakening perspiration easily provoked, sensations of distress about the epigastrium and over the whole abdomen, slow and difficult digestion, abdominal tension, diarrhœa coming and going repeatedly, colic, nausea, hiccough, and at last vomiting. These last symptoms, however, are rare, and do not accompany the evacuations. Thirst also occurs, and desire for acid drinks; fanciful appetite, giddiness, sleeplessness, and tendency to faint. If the disease is limited to these symptoms, convalescence is slow and relapse easily provoked. Moreover, if there is the least imprudence, the invasion of the entire group of characteristic cholera symptoms is prompt.

2. *Algide or Cyanotic Stage.*—Either after the foregoing symptoms, or after prolonged diarrhœa, or after some imprudence, and sometimes without anything of this kind, cholera properly so-called declares itself by sudden illness, with fainting, coincident with vomiting and occurring with evacuations, which become very numerous and follow in quick succession. The evacuated substances resemble milk whey imperfectly clarified, or rice water. They consist of a serous fluid containing floating shreds of coagulated albumen. Soon after painful cramps in the extremities, especially the calves, extending thence over the whole abdomen. The patient complains of excessive pain, burning at the pit of the stomach, intolerable weight about the heart, and insatiable thirst. The anguish is extreme, the voice trembles, the speech of the sufferer is plaintive and jerking. Other secretions—urine, bile, saliva,—are entirely suspended; the evacuations become fætid, the perspiration

also is offensive, indicating approaching death, at the same time animal heat is destroyed. As the pulse sinks, a blue or livid tint (cyanosis) which has commenced at the extremities, extends itself by cold, death-like patches to the entire surface of the body. The nails become blue, almost black; the skin of the fingers is wrinkled, and shrinks on the separate bones of the fingers; the patient becomes so wasted as to be scarcely recognizable. At the same time the eye seems rooted at the base of the orbit, and the upper lid leaves it only half covered. The conjunctiva looks dirty and thick; the cornea is dull and corrugated, as if the eye-ball itself were half emptied; a leaden, turgid look covers the face; the lips become thick and separated; the breath and tongue are cold, and sometimes the nose is so cold as to threaten gangrene. As this terrible scene draws to a close the respiration becomes slow, the muscular tendons twitch, cyanosis covers the body, the patient can no longer swallow, and after a few convulsive movements, he expires.

The intellectual faculties are preserved to the last, but the patient falls into a state of entire apathy, and only wishes to be left to his fate. Attacks of this kind are generally fatal in four to eight hours.

In lighter forms of the attack, the same general group of symptoms is observed, but they follow less rapidly one upon another, and consequently there is more time to meet them. The attack begins with vomiting and diarrhœa; then the loss of vitality and burning at the pit of the stomach; the ejected matter gradually takes the rice-water appearance; the countenance is pinched, the chest contracted; cramps and spasms are excessive; the skin loses all its elasticity; if it is pinched it retains the folding produced; if it is pricked no blood flows, and in twenty-four or thirty-six hours the patient, quite livid, cold, and pulseless, expires in a state of coma.

3. *Stage of reaction.*—If the patient survives the dangers of the preceding period, the graver symptoms lose their

intensity, the spasms and oppression diminish, the natural heat of the body gradually returns, and the pulse steadily resumes its wonted rhythm. At last the evacuations cease, and the suppressed secretions return. The features improve, the patient is able to take some rest, and convalescence is established.

In spite of these favourable signs, precaution must not cease; reaction may either prove abortive, or be exchanged for some grave inflammatory affection. Sometimes the sufferer is carried off by cerebral congestion, or by some inflammation in the respiratory system. More frequently a low or continuous type of fever supervenes, with accelerated pulse and congested features. The patient falls into a state of drowsiness or stupor, the mouth is offensive, there is bilious vomiting. At last the disease ends fatally on the fourth to the eighth day, rarely later, by a typhoid condition.

The indications for our remedies and their various preparations against cholera may be summed up as follows:

1. *Precautions to be observed during the epidemic.*—During the epidemic prevalence of cholera it is most important to take occasional doses of the new Japanese form of scrofoloso, *Scrofoloso giappone.* And as soon as symptoms of diarrhœa set in this remedy should be taken in the first dilution, and continued till the symptoms have subsided, and all tendency to their return has ceased.

Take, dry, 1 globule of S^1 ten or twelve times a day, *i.e.*, about every hour.

In all washing or cleansing operations—in washing the face and hands, &c.—S^1, S^2, or S^5 should be used, in dilution, in the average proportion of 6 globules to a glass of pure water, or water boiled and allowed to cool.

At meal times take, as an habitual drink, spring or filtered water; or boiled water, with good natural wine, if possible, and at the principal meals add 6 or 10 globules of S^1, or of S^1 and L alternately, the first at the midday meal, the last in the evening.

In summer a tepid bath should be taken every three or four days, of thirty or forty minutes duration, medicated by 100 globules of S^5.

2. *Treatment of Cholerine, or incipient Cholera, or of Confirmed Cholera.*—Often an attack may be cut short by 15 or 20 globules of S^1, taken dry and in one dose. Besides this, the patient should drink, in very small and very frequent doses, S^1 dil., either first, second, or third dilution.

Application alternately, every ten minutes, of R. E. and Y. E., or more frequently W. E. and B. E. if the subject is of sanguine temperament, to the pit of the stomach, and to the different centres of the sympathetic nerve as indicated in the plate.

After the attack has yielded, the use of S^1, in first dilution, in small and frequent doses, must be continued for some time, as well as the indicated electricities; and short tepid baths, medicated by 90 or 100 globules of S^5, C^5, or (according to temperament) A^2, with the same number of globules; and rub in unctions of 10 or 12 globules of F^2 over the hypochondria, diluted with a few drops of W. E., and the whole mixed with about 1 oz. of olive oil, which must be shaken whenever it is used.

If the cholera attack is very violent and obstinate, these means must still be persistently used, with the addition, if necessary, of entire tepid baths medicated by a tablespoonful of W. E. or R. E., and frictions all over the body of a liniment composed of 50 or 60 globules of S^5 in half a pint of pure alcohol; also unctions to the hypochondria of F^2, with the same liniment.

All the precautions, and the anti-cholera treatment, which we have just described, may be combined with the ordinary medical instructions issued at these times by sanitary commissioners and boards of health, relating to the medical, hygienic, prophylactic, and curative measures to be taken when this terrible disease makes it appearance. It should be remembered that no rational means of meeting and destroying this malady must be neglected; also that coolness and self-possession should be maintained without flinching in the presence of such a danger. Calm courage, even serenity of mind, a life absolutely sober and regular, are the best aids that can be brought into the service of rational therapeutics.

Infantile Cholera.

Diarrhœa, general sense of illness, depression of strength, tendency to perspiration, sleeplessness, nausea, and then vomiting; water thick, scanty, and high coloured.

Treatment.—The same as the foregoing, in still smaller doses.

Worms.

The disorders produced by worms are many. Different nervous disorders, pains in the stomach, colic, diarrhœa, pallor of the face, sunken eyes, &c. Whenever anomalous symptoms occur, not yielding, or only partially yielding, to the specifics which are indicated, it is right to suspect the presence of worms, especially tœnia, which is the almost invariable cause of these irregular conditions; or the presence of syphilitic virus may be suspected.

This circumstance is justified by the fact that Ver. is invariably useful in all inveterate and obstinate diseases, even cancer; which, although it cannot be directly caused by Entozoa, may nevertheless favour their development.

Worms occupy certain parts of the body and no others; and there are some genera which multiply more than others.

Lumbrici, round worms. *Ascarides lumbricoides* appear especially in weak, lymphatic, scrofulous, badly-nourished children. The chief symptoms are pallor of the face—leaden tint, sunken eyes.

Ascarides, short thread worms; *oxyuris or ascaris vermicularis*, are very small, and are found in the rectum and near the anus.

Tœnia, or tape worm, the long, solitary worm, occupies the small intestine, and may reach the length of thirty or forty feet, or even longer.

In cases of tœnia, the following are the chief symptoms. Sharp or dull colic, tingling and tympanitic or drum-like distension of the abdomen, diarrhœa, white coated tongue, continual expectoration, nausea or vomiting, appetite capricious or absent, sour odour in the breath; face pale and livid, deep sunk eyes, dilated pupils; tendency to rub the nose with the fingers; sleep restless, with grinding of the teeth; pulse irregular and slow; emaciation; urine turbid and milky; sometimes delirium, convulsions, coma, &c.

All these symptoms occur also in the case of lumbrici.

The *tricocephalus*, or longer thread worm, a small, thin worm which inhabits the small intestines, is generally supposed to arise from cerebral causes.

In all worm cases—ascarides, lumbrici, tricocephali, tœnia, and for all the disorders consequent on these parasites, diarrhœa, vomiting, convulsions, epilepsy—the following

Treatment should be pursued. Ver. dil., first or second dilution. The same remedy at meals; and 7 or 8 globules dry at bedtime. Baths of Ver. Unctions, compresses, and enemata of the same remedy. Unctions of F² or of C5 to the hypochondria.

If convulsions, epilepsy, or nervous complications exist, use very feeble doses.

In infants, 2 or 3 globules dry at bedtime.

For tænia. The patient should at first take a decoction of senna, and on the following day begin the use of Ver.

The same process should be repeated for several days till the desired effect, the expulsion of the worms, is produced.

This may occur soon, but after three or four months the symptoms may return: it is therefore necessary to continue treatment till all symptoms have disappeared. The worm is not always expelled bodily. Sometimes it is removed in one piece, sometimes in fragments—in other cases it is absorbed, and the patient is cured, although nothing has been expelled or observed.

Hœmorrhoids: Piles.

Abnormal tumours formed by the dilated veins of the rectum; these tumours often cause an effusion of blood from the rectum or anus, which is termed the hœmorrhoidal flux. Hœmorrhoids are divided into flowing and dry or blind, according to whether they are accompanied or not by the hœmorrhoidal flux, and, according to their seat, they are again divided into external and internal. Different complications may present themselves. Thus, internal hœmorrhoids may fall or be prolapsed, carrying with them a portion of the mucous membrane of the rectum, during defecation. These may be strangulated by sphincter ani, and even become gangrened. Finally, hœmorrhoidal tumours, if they have attained considerable size, are in a continual state of irritation, cause violent pain, threaten to break up, or otherwise degenerate, seriously affecting the general health. Further, the inflammation may spread to the surrounding cellular tissue, and cause abscesses, sloughing of the intestines, fistulas, &c.

Hæmorrhoids are one of the principal indications of the angioitic state, but they sometimes appear in lymphatic subjects with great weakness; in that case they do not bleed, and are not flowing.

Treatment.—For flowing hœmorrhoids, A. in dilution, first dilution. Tepid Sitz-baths, medicated by 50 globules of A^2. For blind hœmorrhoids, S. in dilution, alt. A. Baths of C^5. Unctions of C^5 to the anus.

Prolapsus, or Falling of the Rectum.

Treatment.—C^4 dil., and C^4 dry at meals. C. in dilution, in the second dilution. Baths of W. E., or A^2, or C^5; baths and compresses of C^5, W. E. in compresses. Clysters cold and injections of S^5 or C^5 (10 globules in a glass). Enemata of R. E. (a teaspoonful). Applications of R. E. alt. Y. E. down the dorsal spine, side, and to the perinæum and sacrum.

Prolapsus Ani.

Falling of the lower bowel.

Treatment.—Dil. C., second dilution: baths, unctions, and compresses of C^5. Compresses of W. E. Enemata and washes of C^5. Application of R. E. alt. Y. E. along the dorsal spine, to the ribs and to the perinæum.

Condylomata Ani,

Or fleshy vegetations, always of a syphilitic character.

Treatment.—Dil. Ver. alt. C. Same remedies at meals. Baths of C^5 alt. Ver. Compresses of W. E. Application of R. E. alt. Y. E. along the dorsal spine and to the perinæum. A lengthened treatment must be followed up by S.

RENAL, BLADDER, AND URINARY DISEASES.

Kidneys.

For pains in the kidneys. Dil. S. alt. A^3. The same remedies dry at meal times, 2 to 5 globules. Baths of C^5 alt. S. or of W. E. Unctions and compresses to the renal region of S. or L. Application of R. E. alt. Y. E. to the kidneys, the sacrum, and the dorsal spine.

If the case is that of a woman suffering from leucorrhœa, the treatment is 1 globule dry of S. night and morning, and C. dil., second or third dilution.

In consumptive cases, use the same treatment and add C^5 dil.

Nephritis.

Acute or chronic in the kidneys; dull pain, which becomes continuous and deep, either affecting only one kidney or both, and extending towards the bladder or groin, with red and abundant and turbid urine; loss of appetite, nausea, constipation, fever, disordered digestion.

Treatment.—S. in dilution alt. A^2. Baths of C^5, or W. E. or S^5. Unctions of C^5 or S^5 to the kidneys. Unctions of F^2 or C^5 to the hypochondria. Application of R. E. alt. Y. E. to the occiput, sympathetic, and down each side of the dorsal spine.

Diabetes.

A very serious disease, characterized by an abundant flow of sugary urine; insatiable thirst, enormous appetite, and great emaciation. The most usual termination of the disease is death by exhaustion, or by consecutive disease in the chest superadded to the urinary disorder:—diabetic phthisis.

Food of bad quality or of an exclusively vegetable character, excessive evacuations, fatigue, prolonged watching, moral affections, sadness and fretting, are causes which may favour the development of this disease without necessarily producing it.

Treatment.—Dil. S., 1 globule of L. every hour. Application of R. E. to the solar plexus, sympathetic, the kidneys, the sacrum, and perinæum. Baths of S^5.

In obstinate cases, dil. S. alt. C., or C. alt. A. Baths of C^5 alt. A^2. Application of R. E. alt. Y. E. along the dorsal spine. Unctions of F^2 to the hypochondria and of C^5 to the kidneys.

ALBUMINURIA (*after Nephritis*).

Loss of albumen — which is the most essential constituent of organized bodies—by the urine, attended with pains in the kidneys, and gradual breaking-up of the constitution.

Treatment.—Dil. S. Baths of C^5 or S^5, or A^2 or L. Application of R. E. alt. Y. E. to the sacrum, occiput, and the sympathetic, the whole length of the dorsal spine. Unctions of S^5 to the kidneys. In obstinate cases try C. C^5, S^5, in dilution.

ENURESIS.

This name is given to the involuntary passage of urine.

Treatment.—S. in dilution, or C or A^3, first dilution. 1 globule of C. dry every half hour. Baths of C^5 alt. A^2. Application of R. E. alt. Y. E. to the sacrum and sympathetic. Compresses of C^5 to the pubes; the same of W. E. Unctions of S^5 to the kidney region.

In children enuresis may arise from worms.

Treatment.—Ver^1. 4 globules at bedtime or on waking, Ver., second dilution.

RETENTION (*Ischaria*).

Treatment.—If the patient is sanguine: A^2 dil., second dilution. 1 globule of C^5 every hour. The same remedies at meals. Application of B. E. to the sacrum, the groins, the perinæum, the sympathetic, &c. Baths of L.

If the patient is lymphatic: S. dil., second dilution. The same remedy at meals. 1 globule of C^5 every hour. R. E. applied to the points already enumerated. Baths of L.

INCONTINENCE OF URINE (*Enuresis*).

Treatment.—S. or C. with the application of R. E., and sometimes B. E., to the sympathetic and sacrum.

BLENNORRHAGIA; OR BLENNORRHŒA.

A condition attended with strangury. Acute or chronic discharge from the generative organs: almost always venereal in origin.

Irritating injections and too frequent excitement may produce this, and external treatment is likely to confirm and perpetuate it.

Treatment.—Dil. Ver., or Ver. alt. S. Baths of Ver. alt. S. alt. C5. Injection of Ver. alt. C5.

(*See* general chapter Venereal Diseases).

CYSTITIS.

Acute or chronic inflammation of the membranes of the bladder.

The most notable symptoms of acute cystitis are: constant and severe pain and heat in the hypogastric region; frequent, painful, and often fruitless efforts to urinate; cutting or burning pain during the passage of the water; straining and tenesmus. These symptoms are attended by fever, with much thirst, restlessness, want of sleep. Sometimes there is also hiccough, vomiting, and a urinary odour in the perspiration.

If the water contains mucous, this is not abundant, and is not thick, but reddish.

Acute cystitis generally arises from accidental causes, such as a sudden chill, excess of alcoholic drink, the action of cantharides, badly performed catheterization.

Acute cystitis lasts from ten to twenty days. When it is about to end in resolution, we may see issue, with the water, viscid mucus of a whitish, greyish, or yellowish colour.

Sometimes chronic cystitis follows the acute form, but generally it is not so preceded. Chronic cystitis cannot be regarded as a primary disease; on the contrary, it is generally consecutive upon various pathological conditions of the urinary apparatus and adjacent tissues: and is most usually found in old people.

Its habitual symptoms are: weight and sense of a load at the perinæum; frequent necessity to urinate, which can only with difficulty be accomplished, or which is never satisfying and complete; yellow urine, depositing an abundant mucus, like the white of egg, sometimes also pus or a milky-looking substance; emaciation, yellow tint of the skin, &c.

Treatment.—Dil. F. alt. A. or Ver. second dilution. Unctions of F^2 to the hypochondria. Baths tepid, medicated with C5, S., A^2, or L^2. Compresses of W. E. to the pubes, perinæum and sacrum. Application of R. E. alt. F. to the kidneys, pubes, and sacrum. Unctions of C5 alt. S5 alt. A^2 to the pubic region.

Hœmaturia.

Hæmaturia, or bloody urination, has been divided into renal, vesical, and urethral, according as the blood expelled comes from the kidneys, the bladder, or the urethral canal. Besides this division relating to the seat of the disorder, it is divided into symptomatic and primary hæmaturia.

The most frequent causes of the first are the presence of gravel and calculi in the different parts of the urinary passages, organic lesions of the neck of the bladder, enlargement of the prostate gland, and the forced distension of the bladder by retention of the urine. Hæmaturia occurs also sometimes during scarlatina and grave cases of small pox, in scrofula, &c. It also results from changes in the condition of the blood itself.

Primary hæmaturia, much more rare in our climate than symptomatic, generally follows the suppression of more habitual hæmorrhage; it also occurs sometimes from the abuse of diuretics, from violent purging treatment, the action of cantharides, &c.

Treatment.—S. in dilution alt. A3 second dilution. Unctions on the kidney region and pubes of A. alt. C5; or of A. alt. S5. Baths of L. (100 globules to the bath).

Calculus.

Stony formations in the kidneys, the bladder, or the gall bladder and biliary ducts.

Renal calculi, issuing with the water in the form of gravel; then a greyish or brown stone, with painful micturition, and pains in the loins.

Want of exercise, prolonged continuance in bed, some peculiar formation of the urinary organs, which allows some portion of the fluid to remain behind for some time, may undoubtedly favour the formation of calculus.

If any solid body is by any means introduced into the bladder, whether formed there or brought from without, it inevitably becomes the nucleus of a calculus if it remains.

Calculi may exist for a considerable time and attain a large size before producing any ill effects on the general health. But sooner or later they produce active inflammation in the substance of the kidneys—a condition called nephritic calculus, or nephritis from stone—or they may occasion suppuration and destruction of these organs.

Symptoms.—Lancinating, sharp, and continuous pain in the loins, the bladder, the groin, and the thigh on the affected side, with nausea, vomiting of bile, insomnia, agitation, delirium or convulsions; difficulty in urination.

Under the action of the Mattei remedies the stone is dissolved, and issues in a semi-fluid pasty state, after a continuation of treatment for twenty or thirty days. If the stone is not of the usual lithic character, more time will be required; but in these cases also it is ultimately discharged in the same form.

Treatment.—S. or S. alt. A3, first or second dilution. Baths of S5 and C5. 5 globules of S. at meals. Compresses of W. E. to the pubes, perinæum, and sacrum, Application of R. E. alt. Y. E. to the solar plexus, occiput grand sympathetic, pit of the stomach, and kidney region. Unctions of F^2 to the hypochondria.

DISEASES OF THE SPINE AND SPINAL REGIONS.

Acute and Chronic Inflammation of the Spinal Cord.

Symptoms.—Sharp pains on pressure down the dorsal spine, disordered sensation, convulsive shocks, stiffness, sometimes difficulty in respiration, paralysis of the legs, the bladder and rectum, sharp colic, involuntary evacuations and urination. If the inflammation is near the nape of the neck, the symptoms are: rigidity of the muscles of the neck and arms, tingling or formication in the arms and fingers, very painful respiration. If the inflammation is in the head itself, then: disordered sensation, furious delirium, lockjaw. If it is chronic, the progress of the disease is slower and the symptoms less pronounced. The two forms, acute and chronic, are treated in the same way, except that in the acute form the remedy must be taken in very small and frequent sips, and in very reduced doses.

Treatment.—S. in dilution in the second dilution; with application to the whole of the dorsal spine, the nape of the neck, grand sympathetic, solar plexus, of the electricity most suitable to the temperament of the patient. 1 globule of C^5 every half hour. Baths of W. E. (three tablespoonfuls in each bath). Unctions of C^5 or F^2 to the hypochondria. C. in dilution may also be tried, also S^5, A^2. And in dry globules C^5, S^5, C^4, S^2.

Curvature of the Spine.

This disease is only a form of scrofula.

Symptoms.—Softening and deviation of the bone; swelling of the abdomen; emaciation, weakness, and by contrast enlargement of the head, or of the intellectual faculties.

Treatment.—Dil. S. 10 globules L. at each meal. Baths of S. Bathing all along the spine with brandy containing S., 20 globules to the pint. In obstinate cases dil. A. alt. C. Baths of L. C^5. Application of R. E. alt. Y. E. to the pit of the stomach, occiput, sympathetic, solar plexus, and along the dorsal spine.

Spina Ventosa.

Dilatation of the bone tissues as if blown up by wind, with sharp piercing pains.

Treatment.—C^4 in dilution. Baths of C^4. Compresses of Y. E.

Rickets, Thickening or Curvature of the Bones of the Limbs.

Disorders of rickety children.

Treatment.—S^2 in dilution alt. A. second dilution, or L. in dilution. Alt. C^4 second dilution. Baths of C^4, S^5, of L. or W. E. Applications of R. E. alt. Y. E. to the occiput, sympathetic nerve, solar plexus, and all the nerves related to the affected parts.

Lumbago.

Rheumatism, rendering the patient incapable of bending forwards or backwards, without intolerable pain. This is consequent on a chill.

Treatment.—S. in dilution, first dilution. Baths. Compresses and unctions of C^5. Compresses of W. E. Application of R. E. alt. Y. E. to the sympathetic, occiput, and along each side of the dorsal spine. If there is fever, cut it short with F. in dilution and unctions to the hypochondria of F^2, and follow the above treatment. Some cases of lumbago have yielded to Ver., 10 globules dry at bed time. Ver. in the morning, first and second dilutions.

TORTICOLLIS.

Rheumatism in the muscles of the neck.

Treatment.—This is sometimes removed instantaneously by application of R. E. to the nape. If there is any fever, it should be at once combated by F. A teaspoonful every five minutes for half an hour will often suffice. If this increases the fever, give a weaker dilution, second or third glass. Unctions of F^2 to the hypochondria. If there is no fever, use S. first dilution. Baths of C5. Unctions and compresses of L. Apply R. E. alt. Y. E. to the occiput and sympathetic and to the suffering parts.

CATARRHAL AND PULMONARY DISEASES (*Lung Cases*).

One of the most essential symptoms of lung disease is Cough. We may even call it the pathognomonic, or characteristic or differential symptom of different gradations of morbid condition which may attack the lungs. It is undoubtedly the certain indication of some lesion or obstruction in some part of the respiratory tract. These organs are subject to a great number of inflammatory diseases, on account of the great number of nervous filaments of the pneumogastric nerve, the sympathetic distributed over the tissues, and the very large vascular network which they contain. The nature of the disease depends on the part or tissue affected. Tracheitis is present when the mucous membrane of the fibro-cartilaginous rings of the trachea is attacked; bronchitis, when the corresponding tissues of the bronchial tubes are affected; and pneumonia, when inflammation seizes hold on both the bronchial tubes and the lung substance.

When the case is referable to the connecting cellular tissue, the disease is termed parenchymatous pneumonia. This type of inflammation demands most sedulous precautionary and actual treatment, and persistent use of the indicated specifics. They are required in order to assuage without delay the slow fever which arises, and the insidious inflammatory state which may give occasion to structural changes and degenerations in the lung tissue, and which may be attended with most serious consequences. Sometimes the lung inflammation may remain circumscribed, limited to a single point; but in that case it is deeper. In these cases we often meet with a phlegmonous pneumonia, which is liable to a fatal termination, through the formation of abscess. In other cases it is, on the contrary, more extensive, and then constitutes erysipelatous pneumonia. In these cases the work of the physician is to destroy, as completely as possible, the origin of the disease; else, the spongy and vascular tissues of the lungs may easily keep up, in latent form, an inflammatory germ, which being augmented by internal and external sources of irritation, are liable to manifest themselves unexpectedly in violent ways, and even to lead to very fatal consequences; such as structural changes (tuberculosis, hepatisation), or other not less serious alterations, such as abscess and suppuration in the lung itself.

Cough.

Cough, if taken at the commencement, can be arrested by the following

Treatment.—P. dil. second or third dilution, and some globules given dry every hour. If it is obstinate, compare sections on Lungs, Bronchitis, Laryngitis, &c. Simple catarrh of the chest requires S. alt. P. or P^3; or A. alt. P. or P^3.

Pneumonia.

In pneumonia there is a deep-seated pain, which is usually circumscribed. Respiration may be free and the lung capable of considerable dilatation when the seat of inflammation is the lower part or base of the lungs. But the reverse is the case when the upper lobes are attacked. The patient is able to lie only on the affected side, not on the sound side, without producing pain and cough. We may say it is almost impossible to mistake the diagnosis when there is pulmonary hæmorrhage, and when later on the bloody expectoration takes a rusty coloured tint.

Although less painful than pleurisy, yet this disease produces a pained expression of face peculiar to itself, while in pleurisy the countenance is discoloured by a wine-suggesting redness which is quite *sui generis*. When pneumonia is double, danger is increased in direct proportion to the extent of the lesion and the consequent suspension of the indispensable function of respiration. In these cases the patient is obliged to keep one position, which is generally the sitting attitude.

Pain in the side, which comes on after fifteen or twenty-four hours from the commencement of the attack; at the outset severe and lancinating, in the centre of the breast; oppression; cough; respiration increasing in rapidity. There is difficulty also in breathing; the breathing is short and hurried, cough, viscid transparent expectoration of a reddish or yellowish colour, or sometimes light or dark green, or even, in some exceptional cases, it is white like in a simple cold, and sometimes there is none at all. Fever is high, the tongue coated white, much thirst, headache, urine scanty, and sometimes vomiting.

Treatment.—In the first place, to subdue the fever, F. second dilution, and unctions of F^2 to the hypochondria, afterwards R. E. or B. E., according to the temperament, to the nape of the neck and solar plexus. S. in dilution, alt. P. second dilution, a teaspoonful every five minutes. If the respiration is oppressed, and if there is bloody expectoration, A^3 in dilution, alt. P., alt. S., or alt. C. Unctions C^5 or L. on the chest.

Pulmonary Apoplexy

Is indicated by violent pains in the head; sense of oppression, dull or sharp pains in the chest, and cough with expectoration of dark coloured blood.

Treatment.—The same dry globules as in the preceding case. Dil. A. alt. S. second or third dilution. Application of W. E.

Pleurisy.

In pleurisy the pain is more severe, and shooting and lancinating, more like neuralgia; it is often periodic.

The movements of respiration, and of the chest generally, are effected with pain and difficulty; and in double pleurisy, affecting both sides, as in that which affects only one side, recumbency on the affected side is impossible.

The symptoms of pleurisy, although more marked than those of pneumonia, need not alarm the medical attendant, especially if the disease is recognized as soon as it sets in. When pleurisy is localized, and the lung is not attacked, there is no bloody secretion. It is not unusual for pneumonia to co-exist with and complicate pleurisy: constituting the disease called pleuro-pneumonia.

Treatment.—The same as Pneumonia. Add dry globules of F., five or ten daily.

Gangrene of the Lungs.

This is detected by a special fœtor of the breath, very penetrating, clinging even to the walls of the room. Expectoration of gangrenous masses, diarrhœa, delirium, fever.

The same treatment as the preceding. C. internally and externally.

Pulmonary Phthisis, or Consumption.

Pulmonary disease, and especially phthisis, is found in terrible abundance, and considerably raises the figures of the statistics of death.

This subject is so closely related to the interests of mankind, that I have searched for its most probable causes, and after long and deep study, it seems to me that it is to be found in disturbed equilibrium of cutaneous functions, but principally in a class of causes, the relative influence of which we cannot at present ascertain, causes which influence strongly the general health of individuals, and ultimately of whole nations. As regards disorders of cutaneous function, what can be more anti-hygienic than for a young and delicate woman to have the chest only half covered, dancing a whole evening in rooms so heated as to suggest the temperature of an ante-chamber in the infernal regions. She then goes out with nerves and blood in an ebullition of excitement. She is suddenly exposed to an abrupt stoppage of transpiration, and to those bodily chills which are so well known to every one? What can be said as to certain fashions of treating skin diseases, such as itch, herpetic eruptions, solely by means of external remedies, which force back the secretions upon the mucous membrane of the bronchiæ? Bleeding, also, in phthisical cases, which, while weakening the constitution of the patient, destroys that power of vital resistance by which nature might combat the morbid principles, and which has a strong tendency to damage the tissue of the pulmonary organ? Add to all these causes the disastrous influence of antivenerial treatment, and especially prolonged use of mercurial preparations in strong doses. It is proved that the salts of mercury, and still more metallic mercury itself, affect in a special manner spongy tissues, and consequently, when in the lungs, attack principally the pulmonary substance. We know also that by vital chemic reaction mercury is reduced to its liquid state, as seen in an ordinary barometer, and as it everywhere follows the laws of expansion and contraction existing in the atmosphere, it may, when these oscillations are too violent, cause pulmonary apoplexy, or even phthisis itself. But all these causes of so long standing, and especially those first mentioned, require a more intelligent system of hygiene, and more prudent medical treatment.

One of the most prevalent causes, and one which is much promoted by all civilized governments, is vaccination. It is the sad lot of poor humanity, that the conquests which one day crown it with glory become afterwards instruments of its misfortune and degradation. The immortal discovery of the great benefactor of humanity, Jenner, was soon to become an instrument of homicide, wielded against generations of the human race. Hence, the means has been discovered of founding a sort of *communism* of syphilitic, psoric, scrofulous, and tuberculous inoculation.

Some diseases, like cancer or tuberculosis, which become as it were the *pathologic quarterings* of certain families, traceable in the genealogical line of many direct and collateral branches, mercilessly attack certain victims in whom neither the father, nor mother, nor the immediate ancestors (I am supposing a case where the diseases leave out one generation and reappear in the succeeding one) had ever shown symptoms of this constitution. Besides, how often does it happen that in a numerous family there may be one young man whose thoracic and general formation give no hint of a tendency to phthisis, who, nevertheless, succumbs to this terrible disease, whilst his brothers and sisters do not show the slightest trace of this disorder, and pass through life without showing any tendency to it. Such strange phenomena, which are so constantly to be met with in large centres of population, appear also in new countries, which retain the characteristics of patriarchal types of civilization. The advances made in modern society, the railways, the military system, abolish distance, bring villages and towns into close contact, and establish firm links of connection between the two types of inhabitants. Nowadays, unfortunately, the collective intellectual light which is concentrated in towns, hands on its inheritance of vice to the dwellers in the country, and in this way physical corruption is hourly spread through the land.

In fact, it is easily seen that certain diseases belonging to the lymphatic and circulating systems—humoral diseases—which were at one time restricted to the great centres of population, are now to be found in the most secluded places, hitherto inaccessible. Consequently the recognition of the influence excited by these constitutional principles on the general economy of the body, has become general, with the irresistible extension of scrofulous, ricketty, and other types of disease. The pathologist of to-day knows quite well that scrofula and tuberculosis join hand in hand, and are, indeed, but one and the same potency expressing itself in a thousand different forms of manifestation.

Thus, suppose we vaccinate a number of children, fifteen or twenty, with the vaccine lymph derived from a child whose parents are tainted in their blood by some of the miasmatic influences to which we have referred—suppose, again, that out of these fifteen or twenty children five or six in their turn supply vaccine lymph for a like proportion of other children, it does not require a great stretch of imagination to see what a fearful instrument is at work for the physical degradation of the human race. Let us realize this adequately. In our time humoral diseased forces are only too widely diffused, spite of our fair and prosperous outward seeming, and in general vaccination from infant to infant is a terrible means of propagation. Here is an explanation of the prodigious variety of diseases which are perpetually brought under the observation of practising physicians.

Let medical men consider this, for its importance cannot be overstated, and let governments shake off the apathy with which they have too much ignored these facts; if they wish to have robust soldiers, and vigorous and virtuous citizens, they cannot be indifferent to the *anima sana in corpore sano.* The present practice of vaccination, by means of lymph from arm to arm, used perhaps at the very moment when the child is saturated with the malignant virus of some bad humoral principle, which is therefore in the state in which its poison may be most effectually propagated,—this cannot be accepted with blind acquiescence. Humanity will be a gainer on that day when vaccination with cow-pox virus, taken directly from the calf, is generally adopted. Not that we would attach any severe blame to those who unreflectively practise vaccination, or charge them with wanton blindness. It is not their fault; for in spite of all precautions taken against the spread of diseased humours which are ever increasing in variety in the human race, we cannot avoid constant contact with constitutions thus tainted.

Pulmonary phthisis is caused by the development in the lung of a diseased substance called tubercle.

Symptoms.—At the outset, coldness of the extremities, pallor of the face, hacking cough with expectoration of blood, general *malaise*, appetite lost or morbid; sleeplessness, slight fever, night sweats, great and increasing weakness, emaciation. Afterwards these symptoms become augmented in intensity, and others are added. The expectoration becomes yellow, then greenish, thick, viscid. The chest is contracted, the cheeks hollow, the breathing is oppressed, the legs swollen and puffy.

Treatment.—While the only symptoms are cough and loss of flesh, without sweats, the treatment is S. alt. P.

If oppression of the breath and expectoration of blood declare themselves, we must pursue the treatment by C. Dil. alt. A., alt. P. first or second dilution; then S. dry, night and morning, to restore appetite and produce sleep; for while the pulpy mass of tuberculized lung requires C., the bronchial tubes equally demand P., and the venous system, which is, as well as the bronchial tubes, involved in the pulmonary degeneration, requires the use of A.

The slow fever which always accompanies this disease rarely yields to the febrifuges, but always to A. The dose which is most usually successful is the second dilution. If the purulent expectoration increases, C. must be diminished; if there is a sense of suffocation and nocturnal fever, A. must be given weaker; if cough is severe, P. must be used. An unction of C^5 on the chest relieves pain, and adds to the efficiency of treatment. The application of R. E. alt. Y. E. to the grand sympathetic, to the solar plexus, and the occiput, is important.

Expectoration of Blood.

Under this designation, every kind of bloody expectoration is included, whatever part of the respiratory or digestive tract may be its origin or seat.

Treatment.—Dil. A^3, second or third dilution. If the symptom is in the respiratory tract, A. alt. P. Baths of C^5. alt. A^3. Unctions and compresses at the heart of A^2. Unctions of F^2 to the hypochondria. Application of B. E. to the occiput and sympathetic.

Asphyxia.

Difficult respiration, loss of consciousness, no response to the strongest sensible impression. It may be occasioned by congelation, by submersion, by suffocation, by a fall, by thunder, and by injurious gases.

Treatment.—S. in very strong doses, according to age; 10, 15, or 20 globules dry at once, and repeat according to need till the return of consciousness. R. E. applied to the nape, to the sympathetic, to the occiput, and to the pit of the stomach. Unctions of A^2 to the heart. Similar treatment for oppressed breathing generally.

Asthma.

Spasmodic attack, periodically returning in the respiratory system, characterized by difficulty of breathing; returning at irregular intervals, of varied intensity, without fever. The attack is preceded by yawning, oppression, abundant secretion of urine. This disease is especially dangerous if it proceeds from the chest or the heart. It must be treated especially according to the constitution of the patient; if there is cough, Pettorale should be added.

Treatment.—If the patient is angioitic, Dil. A. second dilution. At the moment of attack, dry globules of S. to cut it short. Application of W. E. to the pit of the stomach, sympathetic, solar plexus. Baths of C5 alt. A2.

If the patient is lymphatic, Dil. S. second dilution. Application of R. E. to the pit of the stomach, sympathetic, and solar plexus. Unctions of C5 to the sympathetic. Baths of L. alt. C5. If there is a catarrhal tendency add Dil. A. alt. P.; or Dil. L. alt. P.

EMPHYSEMA.

Swelling caused by the introduction of air, or the development of gas in the cellular tissue.

Treatment.—Dil. S. or A. In obstinate cases Dil. C. second dilution. Application of R. E. alt. Y. E. to the related nerves.

BRONCHITIS.

Bronchitis is inflammation of the mucous membrane of the bronchial tubes. It is either acute, or chronic, or capillary, or pseudo-membranous.

ACUTE BRONCHITIS.

Symptoms.—Headache, loss of appetite, shivering, pains in the limbs, cold in the head, oppression and pain in the front of the chest, between the breasts; cough aggravated by cold, speaking, movement, occurring in paroxysms, especially evening and night; during these attacks the face becomes red, the eyes water. The attacks sometimes produce vomiting of bilious or viscid mucus, or of food; then expectoration becomes frothy or watery, of a saline taste, sometimes bloody. There is fever and a coated tongue. As bronchitis subsides, the expectoration becomes thicker, and of a greenish or yellow tint.

Treatment.—First of all the fever must be subdued by F. second dilution, and unctions of F^2 to the hypochondria. Then Dil. or P. P^2, or P. alt. F., keeping to the Febrifugos till the fever is subdued. Take care to reduce the doses of the Pectorals if any aggravation of the disease is produced.

If there is blood in the expectoration give daily ¼ of a glass of A. or A^2, in very small doses. Compresses of R. E. or B. E. on the chest are often very beneficial. When the inflammatory stage is past continue the Pectorals, alternately with S.; then S. alone.

Capillary Bronchitis.

Symptoms.—Excessive oppression of the breath; whistling and very hurried respiration, especially in children; cough frequent, causing very severe pain in the chest; expectoration of thready expectoration, frothy, yellow, thick, not giving any relief when ejected. Countenance pale, distressed; speech short and jerking; skin hot, dry, with rapid pulse, lips and cheeks livid; suffocation seems to threaten, and if the disease is not arrested in time, the patient slowly succumbs under advancing asphyxia.

Treatment.—The same as acute bronchitis. Persistent but weak doses of A., and compresses of B. E.

Chronic Bronchitis.

Generally unattended by pain in the chest; simply breathlessness when walking or from slight fatigue. The expectoration is like the white of egg; or else yellow, or greenish, purulent and opaque; cough either frequent or the reverse.

Treatment.—The same as in the acute forms.

Pseudo-Membranous Bronchitis.

This form, which is very rarely met with, is distinguished solely by the ejection, by cough, of false membranes in cylindrical form.

Treatment.—S. alt. A. alt. P.

Hooping Cough.

A convulsive cough in children, and sometimes in adults, occurring in paroxysms. Respiration is difficult, suffocation being threatened, the face congested and livid, the eyes start and water, and the struggle often leads to vomiting.

Treatment.—More cures have been made by A. than by any other remedy. S. and P. may also be tried, or even C., if there is a great abundance of lymph. Whatever be the remedy, it ought generally to be given in the second or third dilution. Unctions of A^2 to the heart. Application of B. E. to the sympathetic.

Simple Laryngitis.

Acute inflammation of the larynx.

Symptoms.—Changed voice, hoarse, shrill voice, sometimes there is aphonia, or loss of voice, burning and pricking in the larynx, painful and difficult deglutition; generally neither fever nor sense of illness; sometimes opaque expectoration.

Treatment.—S. in dilution alt. P. second dilution. If there is fever, F. in dilution, and unctions of F^2 to the hypochondria. Gargles of R. E. and B. E. (one tablespoonful to the glass of water). Unctions of C^5 on the throat.

Chronic Laryngitis.

Not ulcerative.

Symptoms.—The same; little expectoration, but yellowish, and especially in the morning.

Treatment.—S. in dilution alt. P. Baths of C5. Unctions and compresses of C5, and S5, and B. E.

Chronic Ulceration of the Larynx.

Symptoms.—The same, but with purulent or bloody expectoration; offensive breath, evening fever, and night perspirations, increasing cough, almost always the accompaniment or premonition of pulmonary phthisis supervening on existing tuberculosis.

Treatment.—S. in dilution alt. A. alt. C. Discontinue A. when the expectoration of blood ceases. If phthisis is present P. alt. A^3 alt. C5 second or third dilution. Unctions of C5 over the chest. Gargles of R. E. (one teaspoonful to the glass of water). Unctions of A. to the heart. Application of B. E. to the grand sympathetic and solar plexus.

Syphilitic Laryngitis.

The consequence of a recent or distant, often distant, affection of the same kind contracted during youth, and believed to be cured.

Treatment.—For one or two months, Ven. in dilution alt. S. The same remedies alternated at meal time (from 5 to 10 globules). Then S., and if the case is obstinate P. alt. A^3 alt. C5.

In all these cases, the application of W. E. or B. E. may be of much service. The internal remedies must also be given in gargles at least twice a day.

Croup.

True croup comes on very gradually and slowly. The first attack generally comes in the day. It is epidemic.

The cough is hollow, raw, and muffled. Shreds of membrane are thrown out by cough and vomiting.

Sharp pains in the larynx and the back of the throat. The voice is whistling; and generally there is aphonia, loss of voice; there is fever; and the symptoms are unintermittent. The disease is inflammatory.

Treatment.—Calm the feverish state by F., third dilution, and unctions of F^2 to the hypochondria. Then Dil. of S. alt. P. alt. A^3 second dilution, every five minutes a teaspoonful, 1 globule of S. every five minutes. Gargle with S., 15 globules to the glass of water, or with B. E., 20 drops to the glass. Unctions of C^5, and application of R. E. to the throat, and to the great sympathetic between the shoulders.

False Croup

Comes on suddenly, and in the night; it is not epidemic; the cough is dry, resounding, sonorous, without expectoration,—there is little pain in the larynx; the voice is hoarse, hollow, or barking, but distinct. There is no fever.

Treatment.—The same as for true croup.

Aphonia.

Disease of the respiratory system, producing a partial or total loss of voice. This affection is symptomatic of other diseases. Inflammation of the larynx, the stomach, the bronchial tubes, the lungs. Worms, pregnancy, any great chill, skin disease, suppressed hœmorrhage, and latent syphilis may be causes. It is easily cured when it results from suppressed skin disorder or hœmorrhage.

Treatment.—Dil. A. alt. S. Same remedies at meals. Gargles of W. E. Baths of C^5 alt. A^2. Application of R. E. to the occiput, sympathetic, solar plexus, and pit of stomach; sometimes R. alt. Y. E. to the hypochondria.

COLD, AND ITS CONSEQUENCES, CHILL.

In the first place, the fever must be suppressed by F. Dil. first or second dilution. Dil. S^2, first glass. Unctions of C^5 to the hypochondria. Compresses of W. E. to the head.

Treatment.—P. in dilution, second dilution. Gargles of R. E., or B. E. Applications of R. E., alt. Y. E. to the occiput, large and small hypoglossi. Baths of C^5. If the case is obstinate, P. in dilution, alt. S., or P. alt. C^5.

INFLUENZA.

The symptoms are those of simple bronchitis with catarrh.

Symptoms.—Cold in the head, fever, headache, heaviness in the limbs, excessive weakness, loss of appetite; dry, difficult, and painful cough, provoking later on a more or less abundant mucus expectoration. According to the temperament of the individual, nervous symptoms are developed, as: delirium, starting, twitches, great exhaustion, &c.

Treatment.—At the commencement the fever must be cut short by the use of F^1 second dilution, to be taken in frequent and small sips. Compresses of F^2 to the hypochondria. Gargles with R. E. or W. E. or B. E. (10 or 20 drops to the glass of water). Then P^1 or P^3 in dilution, second dilution, and finally S. Unctions of C^5 on the chest. Application of R. E. or B. E. on the chest.

DISEASES OF THE HEART AND CIRCULATION.

HEART.

The cavities of the heart, the veins and arteries, being continually in contact with the blood, which is, so to speak, one of the factors of inflammation, are necessarily exposed to inflammatory seizures, as one may ascertain by daily observation. The angioitics promptly destroy these inflammatory centres, so that a function of such importance as the circulation need never be disturbed, but follow its normal course without interruption. This is a most important consideration, since any disturbance in the circulation is capable of giving rise to still more serious disorders, dangerous to life itself.

The characteristic marks of heart disease consist in irregular action or pulsation of this organ. There is increased activity of the contractile force, manifested by cardiac palpitation. Sometimes, on the other hand, there is diminished force, producing an abated or lowered circulation. Also the functions of the heart may be changed in quality, and intermittent action then arises.

The most notable inflammatory disorders of the heart are: *pericarditis*, inflammation of the investing membrane, or that which covers the heart; *carditis*, or inflammation of the substance of the heart; *endocarditis*, or inflammation of the interior living membrane of the heart.

By the aid of differential diagnosis these affections may be recognized and distinguished from one another. This distinction, however, is needless, if our therapeutic resources are employed, since all these diseases require the use of the angioitics.

However, we may summarily indicate the different symptoms of acute diseases of the centre of circulation. The patient complains of a sharp, almost burning, pain near the xyphoid cartilage, the end of the breast bone—rather to the left than the right; that is to say, in the precardial region, whence it radiates in different directions. Considerable oppression in breathing, not at all arising from pulmonary disease, since percussion and auscultation do not reveal the least trace of pneumonia or pleurisy; alteration of expression; short and rapid breathing, but without mucus rale; cough accompanied by mucus expectoration; violent and often irregular action of the heart;

a pulsation scarcely perceptible, but more frequent and sometimes intermittent. The patient prefers to lie on his back, with head raised; it is impossible for him to lie on the cardiac side of the body, for this position makes the pain more intense. He finds absolute repose essential, since the least movement augments his pain. Besides these symptoms others are present, which are, so to speak, the offspring of the first; such as delirium, intolerable anguish, subsultus and starting of the tendons, hiccough, great difficulty in swallowing, vomiting, swelling of the joints, frequent fainting, often a want of correspondence between the arterial pulse and the action of the heart. The pathognomonic or differential symptom of cardiac disorders, which consist in neuralgic pain going from the neck to the shoulders and the interior side of the left arm, attains the highest intensity.

In pathological conditions of the heart, it is well to administer A. in very small doses, second or third dilution, at short intervals; *i.e.* a teaspoonful every three or four minutes; taking care to add light use of B. E. When the symptoms become less violent the dose may be gradually augmented.

The action of the angioitics is admirably exhibited in inflammations of the heart, the arteries, and the aorta. All disorders of the great arteries find, in the angioitics, remedies which entirely supersede bleeding, leeches, and the enormous doses of digitalis employed by ordinary physicians, the disastrous consequences of which are well known.

Hahnemann, whose observing faculty nothing escaped, had in his time observed the sad results of the abuse of digitalis in diseases of the heart. The valves of the heart remain congested or paralyzed ; the action of the valves is enfeebled ; a general condition of disorder is spread over the whole of the functional action of the organ, and it is not possible to reckon with any confidence on the recovery of any patient who has tried digitalis for any length of time in order to relieve slight cardiac disturbance or palpitation.

Pericarditis, or excessive secretion of serous fluid in the pericardium (dropsy of the pericardium, or hydropericarditis) requires both the external and internal use of the angioitics. They are also very useful in the cases of syncope or fainting, provided always they do not proceed from any organic disease of the heart or its valves: in this case they are only palliatives. Equally necessary are angioitics in the treatment of hypertrophy, aneurism of the heart or of the large arteries. They are efficacious in case of pulsation of the celiac or epigastric artery, which is often felt at the pit of the stomach, and which almost always accompanies an attack of gastritis: in stenocarditis or neuralgia of the heart; in certain cardiac neuroses produced by moral causes or repeated misfortune; against sudden waking with convulsive starts when lying upon the left side, if this symptom does not arise from organic mischief; lastly, in all diseases of the veins, in varices, and the hœmorrhage from varicose ulcers. Not only are they sovereign in inflammation of the arteries, but also in phlebitis, or inflammation of the veins. However, when phlebitis attacks the uterus, it is right to use the cancerous remedies in alternation with the angioitic.

External treatment in disorders of the heart is of the first importance. It is to be well noted that a diseased heart must always be treated with very minute doses, especially when there are indications of dilatation.

Treatment.—The general remedy in heart cases is A. in very small doses, second or third dilutions, and at first only a few teaspoonfuls daily. Compresses of A. (15 or 20 globules to the glass) are most essential parts of treatment; they should be often changed.

Light application of B. E., for only two or three seconds, removes palpitation. In some cases a few globules of A. dry, have been attended with the best possible results.

Hydropericarditis.

Dropsy of the investing serous membrane of the heart.

Treatment.—A^2 alt. C^2 second or third dilution sipped frequently. Baths of A^2 and C^5. Unctions of F^5, on the hypochondria. In case of violent palpitations, the hand moistened with several drops of B. E. should be passed rapidly over the heart.

Aneurism

Is a tumour formed in the course of an artery by dilatation of its coats. It indicates an angioitic temperament, and is attended by oppressed breathing, cerebral congestion, sometimes cough. A tumour external to the artery, but at the seat of the aneurism, may be present, and this. is always the seat of pulsation and throbbing. The weakened heart must be treated by the feeblest possible doses, a few teaspoonfuls daily being all that is at first required. Aneurisms require external rather than internal treatment.

Treatment.—If there is violent palpitation, the hand, moistened with a few drops of B. E. should be passed gently over the tumour or the heart.

Compresses of A^2 or A^3 (20 globules to the glass) on the heart are essential in the treatment.

Dilution of A. second or third dilution, a few teaspoonfuls daily. Application over the heart for a few seconds at a time of B. E.

Angina Pectoris.

A kind of pulmonary suffocation, appearing suddenly by a sense of illness and restlessness, sharp suffocating pains in the upper front part of the chest, extending to the left shoulder and the arm, and extending into the limbs as numbness, formication, a creeping sensation followed by an indescribable physical languor or sense of exhaustion. The disease may arise as much from nervous perturbation as from alteration of the sanguinary system.

Treatment.—Dil. S. alt. P.; or C. alt. P. Gargles of R. E. or of C^5. Unctions of C^5 all over the chest. Compresses of A^2 to the heart.

DISEASES OF THE GENERATIVE ORGANS.

For fuller and additional particulars, see general chapter on Venereal Diseases.

Hydrocele.

Hydrocele is the effusion of serum into the investing sheath and substance of the testicle, and into cellular tissue of the scrotum.

Treatment.—S^5 alt. C^5. Application of R. E. to the sacrum and perinæum. Compresses of F^2 to the hypochondria. Enemata with 20 globules of C^5. Baths of L.

Impotence.

Incapacity of generative function. Powerlessness in either sex resulting from: sometimes, (1) some perceptible organic defect; or, (2) disease in the generative organs; (3) exhaustion of strength. It is characterized less by the impossibility of intercourse in the ordinary way, than by the impossibility of fertile union.

Treatment.—S. in dilution, or A., according to temperament; which should be alternated with C. Application of R. E. alt. Y. E. to the grand sympathetic, occiput, solar plexus, pit of the stomach, sacrum, and perinæum. Baths medicated by three tablespoonfuls of W. E., or R. E., or B. E.

Masturbation.

Voluntary and involuntary. Sometimes caused by the presence of worms.

Treatment.—S. in dilution alt. C., or S. alt. Ver. Application of R. E. to the occiput, sympathetic, and sacrum; 1 globule of C5 every half hour. Compresses of W. E. to the occiput. If caused by worms, take 10 globules of Ver. Baths of S5. 3 drops of Y. E. on sugar.

Spermatorrhœa.

Dil. S. alt. A. or A3 second dilution. The same remedies at meals. Baths of L. or C5. Unctions of F2 to the hypochondria. Some drops of B. E. taken internally on sugar. Application of R. E. alt. Y. E. to the six chief centres. W. E. to the sacrum, pubes, and perinæum.

Uterine Disease.

The uterus, the most impressionable organ in women, is often the cause of physical and moral disorders. (*See* Insanity, Leucorrhœa, Hysteria, Epilepsy, Metritis).

Uterine Pains.

Treatment.—5 globules of C. dry are often all that is necessary. C. in dilution, first dilution. Baths of C5. Unctions and compresses of C5 to the pubes. Compresses of W. E. to the sacrum. Application of R. E. alt. Y. E. to the sacrum and sympathetic.

Prolapsus Uteri

May be complete or incomplete. Patients suffering from simple relaxation have the following symptoms: dragging and bearing-down pains in the back and groins; difficult digestion; constipation, with feeling of weight in the anus; pain in the stomach; frequent urging to urination or urinary retention; leucorrhœa; more or less inflammation of the uterus and vagina. In complete falling of the womb the symptoms point to deeper irritation and more intense inflammation. The parts must be inspected to ensure a perfect diagnosis.

Treatment.—C. in dilution or C. alt. A., first dilution, or C^5, first dilution. Same remedies dry at meals. Baths of C^5 alt. A^2. Unctions and compresses of C^5 to the pubes, perinæum, and sacrum. Injections of C^5 and W. E. (one tablespoonful to a pint of water). Applications of R. E. alt. Y. E. to the pubes and sacrum. In some cases pieces of linen soaked in W. E., and introduced into the vagina, has proved successful.

Puerperal Metritis.

Inflammation following upon accouchement.

Treatment.—C. in the second dilution. 1 globule of C^5 every half-hour. Unctions and compresses of C^5 to the stomach and pubes. Application of R. E. alt. Y. E. to the saerum.

Leucorrhœa.

A whitish, yellowish, grey, or rose-coloured discharge, thick or watery, with or without odour, from the vagina or vulva. This discharge is accompanied by paleness of the face, griping pains in the stomach, difficult digestion, palpitation and breathlessness in walking, irregular or suspended monthly flow, headache, &c.

Treatment.—C. in dilution, second or third dilution. The same remedy at meal times. 1 globule of C^5 every hour. If there is constipation, C. alt. S. second dilution, or C. alt. A^3. In obstinate cases A^2. alt. C^5. 1 globule of C. every hour. If these small doses do not diminish discharge, it may be presumed that worms are interfering with the treatment. In this case 8 or 10 globules of Ver. may be given at night, at bedtime, and, in the morning, second dilution of Ver. alt. A.

Vaginitis.

Chronic or acute inflammation of the mucous membrane of the vagina.

Treatment.—C. dil. or C5 second dilution. The same remedies at meals. Baths of C5. Compresses of C5 to the pubes, the perinæum, and the nerves of the sacrum.

Ovaritis.

Inflammation of the ovaries.

Symptoms.—Pain in the uterine region, with swelling on one side, extending into the groin and thighs, obstinate constipation. This inflammation is accompanied by enlargement and dropsy of the ovary.

Treatment.—A. alt. with C. in second dilution. 1 globule of C5 every hour. Unctions and compresses of C4 on the painful parts. Application of R. E. alt. Y. E. to the sympathetic, solar plexus, and down the dorsal spine. Injections of C5.

Polypus in the Uterus.

Treatment.—C. alt. A2 in second dilution. 1 globule of C4 every hour. Baths of C5. Unctions and compresses of C5 alt. A2. In case of hæmorrhage injections of A3. Application of R. E. alt. Y. E. to the sacral nerves.

Chronic Congestion, Induration, Granulation, or Ulceration.

C. alt. S. in the second dilution. 1 globule of C5 every hour. Baths of C5. Unctions and compresses of C5 to the pubes. Application of R. E. alt. Y. E. to the sympathetic, solar plexus, and down each side of the dorsal spine. Injections of C5.

Hæmorrhage from the Uterus.

(*See* Menstruation.)

Cancer of the Uterus.

(*See* Cancer.)

Nymphomania.

Intense uterine excitement.

Treatment.—C. in dilution or C5 in the second or third dilution. 1 globule of C5, dry, every half hour. Lotions of C5 to the pubes and sacrum. Application of W. E. to the sympathetic, solar plexus, nape of the neck, and sacral nerves.

Gangrene of the Uterus.

Occurring after accouchement. The symptoms are those of inflammation of the uterus; fœtid discharge, violent fever, pallor, pain in the groins, in the lower part of the abdomen, the sacrum, and the kidney region. Marked disease like distension. The pain disappears when the gangrene is advanced.

The same treatment, with injections of C5 (25 globules to a glassful of water).

It has been observed by the most eminent physicians that gangrene may arise from congestion of the arteries near the part attacked, or near a part in connection with the part attacked.

This cause suggests that the addition of A. in the treatment of gangrene may lead to good results.

Menstruation.

Excessive menstruation; menorrhagia.

Treatment.—It is to be remembered that the angioitics in ordinary doses bring on the monthly period, while at the second dilution they moderate it, or suppress it altogether.

Menstrual Spasms or Dysmenorrhœa.

Treatment.—These are almost always suppressed by 2 globules of C. In obstinate cases the dose should be repeated every half-hour. Application of W. E. Unctions of C5 over the uterus and ovarian regions.

Amenorrhœa.

Caused by a chill. It consists in absence, suppression, or great diminution of the monthly flow.

Treatment.—Dil. C. alt. A., second dilution. Baths, injections, compresses of C5 or A2. Application of R. E. alt. Y. E. to the sacrum, and the whole length of the dorsal spine. Light application of B. E. over the heart. Dry globules of the same remedies at meals.

Dysmenorrhœa.

Pain and difficulty in the monthly period.

Treatment.—A3 alt. C5, first dilution, and 5 globules of the same remedies, *alternately*, at meal times.

Critical Age.

That period in woman's life when menstruation ceases. This crisis is also called the menopause; it comes at the age of 45 or 50. It is the general impression that the early appearance of the menstrual flux indicates a liability to have many children. The cessation of the menses may produce various accidents, and at this age more than ordinary care should be taken of the general health.

Treatment.—Dil. S., sometimes A. Same remedies at meals. Baths of C5 (100 globules). Injection of A. (20 globules to a tumblerful of water).

Accouchement.

Any woman who wishes to secure a safe and easy confinement ought not to omit taking, during pregnancy, dil. S.; injections occasionally of C5., 15 globules in about 8 ounces of water; and a bath once a week, with 50 globules of C5.

Difficult Labour.

Treatment.—C1 in dilution, second dilution, or 1 globule of C5, dry, every hour. Application of W. E. to the sacrum.

Arrested Labour

Arises from uterine spasms, specially at the neck of the uterus; or from inertia.

Treatment.—Dil. C., 10 globules of S. or of C5, dry. Application of R. E. alt. Y. E. to the sacrum and sympathetic.

False Pregnancy.

Dropsy or gaseous distension of the uterus are not false pregnancies, but simply liquid or gaseous accumulation.

False pregnancy exists when an undeveloped germ takes on an irregular or incomplete development; sometimes there is only a development of a thready placental fringe; sometimes the fœtus is expelled, and a rudimentary organization of the placenta, and then a growth of the uterine mucous membranes.

Treatment.—Dil. S. alt. C. Baths of C5. Unctions over the abdomen of C5. Application of R. E. and Y. E. to the sacral nerves and the sympathetic. 1 globule of S. every hour.

Abortion.

Premature expulsion of the fœtus, without the placenta, and before its full development, constitutes abortion.

A plethoric habit, or an anœmic, nervous state in the woman; some severe attack, such as fainting, small-pox, lead colic, bodily distortion, syphilis, too heroic administration of mercury, placental apoplexy, detachment of the placenta, strong excitement, moral or physical disorders in the abdominal organs, uterine debility, or heightened sensibility of this organ, the presence of twins or more than two, the death of the fœtus, rupture of the cord, accident or violence—these are causes likely to produce abortion.

When it arises from a faulty constitutional state it always occurs at the period corresponding to the monthly flow.

Abortion at first pregnancy, not occasioned entirely by

traumatic or accidental causes, is liable to lead to a tendency to abortion in subsequent pregnancies.

Preventive Treatment.—Dil. S. alt. A^3, alt. C^5. Baths of A^3 and C^5.

Stérility or Barrenness.

Usually caused by some disease of the uterus, indicated by whites, or leucorrhœa and other symptoms; disappearing by the cure of this organ.

Treatment.—C. dil. second or third dilution. Injections of C^5 into the vagina. Unctions of C^5 on the sacrum.

Breast.

Ulcerations, cracks, or chaps, and inflammations in the breast are treated by C. dil. or C^2 alt. A. second dilution. Baths and compresses of C^5.

For tumours, discharges, abscesses, and all maladies of the breast, we may always start with C. internally, and C^5 externally.

Milk.

Milk fever; suppression of the milk.

Treatment.—C. in dilution or C^5, second dilution. Compresses of W. E. on the breast. R. E. alt. Y. E. to the grand sympathetic, solar plexus, and pit of the stomach.

Galactorrhœa.

Flow of milk from the breasts when nursing is not proceeding.

Treatment.—C. in dilution alt. A. second dilution. The same remedies at meal times (from 5 to 10 globules). Baths of C^5 or W. E. 1 globule of C^5 every hour, or 20, dry, on waking. Applications of R. E. or Y. E. to the occiput and solar plexus.

Aversion

Of the infant to nursing; should be treated by giving to

the nurse S^2; to the infant unctions of C^5 to the hypochondria, and some teaspoonfuls of S^1 in the third dilution.

Alba Dolens,

Or white leg, is a disease peculiar to women after confinement. It is indicated by white swelling, with heat on the surface, in one or both of the lower limbs. If badly treated it may last for a year. There may or may not be fever.

Treatment.—If there is fever A. alt. F^1 second dilution. Unctions of F^2 to the hypochondria. Compresses of A^3 on the affected veins. Compresses of B. E. Application of B. E. to the sympathetic.

SKIN DISEASES.

Skin.

It must be remembered that for all diseases of the skin S., and especially S^5, is pre-eminently the remedy. Ulceration, not arising from very grave disorganization of the lymph or blood, or from a cancerous diathesis, is rapidly cured by:—

Treatment.—S. in dilution or S^5, S. alt. A^3. Baths of S^5, and compresses of C^5.

Eruptions.

All cutaneous disorders, erythema, erysipelas, roseola, herpes, eczema, impetigo, urticaria or nettlerash, lupus, psoriasis, and itch, yield to the following

Treatment.—S. in dilution, second dilution. Baths of S^5, and compresses of R. E. alt. Y. E. Scrofoloso, when taken in strong doses, has a powerful effect in dispersing skin eruptions. It is useful to know this in the case of repercussed eruption during eruptive fever, but is useless for purifying the blood. For a simple eruption S. is given in small doses.

Acne.

Isolated, pointed pustules, slightly suppurating, on the nose, the cheeks, sometimes the back, leaving persistent livid blotches which reappear and disappear rapidly.

Coppery pimples and mentragra are varieties. This eruption is especially apt to appear in plethoric persons, subject to hæmorrhage, which has been partially or entirely suppressed; in women at the critical age, and in persons with high colour, addicted to good living and alcoholic drinks.

Treatment.—Dil. S. second dilution. Sometimes A. alt. S. Baths of S5 or C5. Application of R. E. alternately with Y. E. to the solar plexus, the pit of the stomach, the sympathetic at the stomach, occiput, and cervical centre.

If the acne is syphilitic, dil. of Ven. or C5 alt. Ven.; sometimes baths of A2 must be added; or alternate baths of Ven. C5 and A2. The remedies also should be alternated at meals.

Eczema.

Eruption of a number of small vesicles collected together, forming large and irregular patches, from which flows a serous discharge, producing excoriation of the skin, and intolerable itching, which is aggravated by the heat of the bed. It is not contagious.

These vesicles, at first transparent, then turbid, are of different sizes. When they break the contained fluid dries and forms crusts or yellow scabs.

Treatment.—This is cured by S. or by S. alt. A., in ordinary doses. In obstinate cases, C., or 1 globule of C5 every hour. Compresses of S5. Unctions of S. on the parts, and of F2 to the hypochondria. Baths of L.

The most usual treatment is as follows: Dil. S. second dilution, or of S. alt. A. The same remedies in the wine taken at meals, and 1 globule of C5 every hour. Baths of

S^5 alt. C^5. Compresses of C^5 to the hypochondria. Application of R. E. alt. Y. E. to the occiput, the great sympathetic, and solar plexus. 10 globules of S^5 to the ounce of Cerate, and some drops of R. E., for a pomade to apply every evening on the parts where eczema prevails.

Intertrigo.

An irritation of the skin resulting from excoriation. In infants and small children it is often the result of neglected wetting.

Treatment.—S. in dilution, second dilution. Compresses of W. E. Washing with C^5, 20 globules in a quart of water. If there is bleeding, compresses of A.; not bleeding, compresses of S. If on the genitals, Ven. internally and externally. Baths of C^5. Application of R. E. alt. Y. E. to the sacrum.

Scabies (Itch).

Eruption of little transparent vesicles between the fingers, on the thumbs, always appearing on the side of the arm which touches the body when it is hanging free, inside the thighs, and in the bendings of the joints of the limbs. It is well-known that it is contagious, and is accompanied by much irritation.

Treatment.—S. in dilution alt. A. second dilution. Baths of C^5, S^5, A^3, W. E. Unctions of F^2 to the hypochondria. Applications of R. E. alt. Y. E. to the grand sympathetic and solar plexus.

S. expels the itch, and after eight days it dries up. The treatment must be continued; after a few days the disorder reappears; this is repeated two or three times, after which it disappears entirely, proving that the blood is restored to its natural state.

Pruritus.

With eruption of small pimples.

Treatment.—Dil. A. alt. S. Same remedies at meals. Baths of C^5, F., A^2, or L. Application of R. E. alt. F. to the sympathetic, occiput, solar plexus.

Impetigo.

Eruption of small pustules, which, on becoming dry, are transformed into semi-transparent pale yellow crusts; they are scattered or collected.

For treatment, *see* Lupus.

Facial Impetigo.

A scabby eruption of chronic type, consisting of pustules more or less detached, which suppurate, forming large semi-transparent crusts. When dry, they form hard ridges, very thick, and of a yellow-greenish colour.

Same treatment as Lupus.

Milk-Scab.

Eruptions in nursing children.

Treatment.—S. in dilution should be given to the nurse, and 1 globule of C^5 every hour. Unctions of C^5 to the part affected.

Serpiginous Crusts.

The nurse must have 1 globule of S. dry every half-hour. Unctions of C^5 or S^5 on the child's head.

Tinea or Favus.

An eruption on the hairy scalp, taking the form of dull coloured, dirty-looking scab, more moist at the centre than at the circumference, a small margin, and depressed surface.

Treatment.—S. dil. In obstinate cases S. alt. C., or S. alt. A. second dilution. Baths of S^5 or C^5. To the eruption apply compresses of S^5 or C^5 or L. Baths of L.

Erysipelas.

Vulgarly called St. Anthony's fire, with a more or less vivid redness of the skin, and a certain amount of hardness and tumefaction in the affected part. The precursors of erysipelas are: Sense of illness, lassitude, fever, nausea, headaches (which are severe if the disease is on the face). Then, on the appearance of erysipelas, there may be a high fever, shiverings, thirst, vomiting, agitation, and even delirium, diarrhœa, or very tenacious constipation. It may end in resolution, desquamation, suppuration, and sometimes gangrene.

Treatment.—S. in dilution, or A., or A. alt. S., according to the constitution. Applications of R. E. or B. E. to the corresponding nerves.

In violent erysipelas of the face R. E. should be applied to the nape of the neck, and each side of the atlas in the nape of the neck. Compresses of S. (20 globules in a glass) on the erysipelas have also given quick results. At the commencement it can be prevented by repeated applications of R. E. to the occiput, to the supra- and infra-orbital regions, and to the sympathetic nerve, or with W. E., or B. E., or R. E. alt. Y. E.

Phlegmonous Erysipelas

In the arm, accompanied by vertigo.

Treatment.—A. in dilution, second dilution. Baths of C5. Compresses of W. E. or A.

Periodical Erysipelas.

Treatment.—F. in dilution alt. A2. Baths of C5. Unctions of F2 to the hypochondria. Compresses of A2.

Erysipelas with Œdema in the Lip.

S. in dilution alt. A. Baths of C5 alt. A2. Unctions and compresses of C5 alt. A2. Unctions of F2 to the hypochondria.

Ecthyma.

Eruption of rounded pustules, suppuration, with a hard and inflamed base ; followed by a more or less thick scab which becomes brown, and leaves a reddish stain on the skin.

Acute ecthyma is always attended by some degree of fever, which gives it the character of a specific eruptive fever.

Treatment.—Dil. S. or Ven. second or third dilution. The same remedies at meal time. Baths of S^5 and C^5. Compresses of S^5 on the suffering part. Application of R. E. alt. Y. E. to the occiput, the solar plexus, the pit of the stomach, and the great sympathetic. Unctions of F^2 to the hypochondria.

Elephantiasis.

A disease of the lymphatic vessels, characterized by hard and permanent swelling, which is limited at first to the lymphatic vessels of the affected parts, but becoming gradually general. There is no organ which is not exposed to the attack of this disease, but the limbs, especially the lower limbs, are most liable. As a rule it appears on only one side of the body.

The causes of elephantiasis are very obscure. It is frequent in the tropics, and rare in our own latitudes. It is neither hereditary nor contagious.

The first attack of this malady is marked by a fixed pain in a knot of glands or in the course of the lymphatic vessels. To this pain there is added redness, and hard swelling, unequal and nodulated. Sometimes movement is impeded in the part attacked. It is tender to pressure, a febrile condition follows, and lasts for twenty-four hours. Swelling remains only during nine days, and then disappears.

The same phenomena reappear at more or less remote intervals.

At each recurrence the swelling becomes harder and more persistent for a long time. At last it becomes continuous. It then increases during the attacks, and diminishes when they have ceased.

This disease is only fatal in cases in which the changes in the cutaneous tissues are carried to internal organs.

Treatment.—Dil. S. alt. A. second or third dilution. Baths of L., S5, C5, A3. Compresses of G. E. covered with larger compresses of S5 alt. A3. Application of R. E. alt. Y. E. to the related nerves, to the occiput, the sympathetic, the solar plexus. Unctions of A3 to the heart, and of F2 to the hypochondria. Try C2 in dilution.

Ichthyosis.

Under this head are comprised certain disorders where the skin is covered with dry, white, and imbricated scales, with lumps in the form of horns and claws; or it becomes rough and wrinkled. These disorders are endemic in certain places; the causes are very obscure.

Treatment.—A1 in dilution alt. C1 second dilution. Baths of C5. 10 globules of S1 every morning dry on the tongue.

Patches.

Discolouration of the face in patches; wine-coloured marks.

Treatment.—A. dil. or A2 second dilution. Baths of A2. Compresses of A2 alt. B. E. to the affected part. Unctions of A2 to the heart.

For hepatic patches, F. dil. second dilution. Baths of C5 alt. W. E. Unctions to the hypochondria of F2 or C5.

Panaris, or Whitlow.

Treatment.—At the beginning it may be cut short by: Compresses of R. E., or of W. E., or of C5. If at the commencement it cannot be stopped, treat with S. in dilution alt. C^5, in the second dilution. Compresses of S^5 or A^2. Baths of C^5. Take 5 globules of S^5 alt. C^5 in wine at meal times.

Whitlow has been averted and cured in two days by holding the finger for some time in W. E. or Y. E., and wrapping it up at night in compresses of the same electricity.

Ecchymosis,

I.e., dark or bluish patches of skin, owing to an accumulation of blood in the sub-cutaneous cellular tissue; from bruises or contusions.

Treatment.—Dil. A. second dilution. Compresses of A^2, of C^5, of B. E., or W. E., on the affected parts.

Stings of Insects.

When the wound is dark or livid, especially from a wasp or hornet, C. must be used internally and externally. As soon as the gangrenous appearance has subsided the treatment should be concluded by S.

Bee Stings

Are treated by Dil. F. alt. S. Compresses of R. E. alt. Y. E.; the last by cupping.

Splinters.

Small wooden spiculæ accidentally introduced into the substance of the skin, which determine by their presence severe irritation, and often very serious consequences.

Treatment.—Steep the part in a warm bath, medicated by 25 drops of R. E. to each glass; then dilution of S. After half an hour passed in the bath, the splinter may be easily removed.

Chilblains.

An ailment resulting entirely from cold, and especially

from exposure of cold parts to very strong heat. Occurs most often in children, in persons of a lymphatic temperament, or of a delicate and scrofulous constitution.

Treatment.—S. in dilution, with compresses on the related nerves of R. E. or W. E., a dilution of A^2. Compresses and unctions of A^2. A certain cure results from a pomade of A, 10 globules to the ounce of Cerate and 10 drops of B. E. The chilblains must be rubbed with the ointment, and wrapped up during the night. After several days they will disappear.

Lepra.

This disease is characterized by hard and fine and non-sensible tubercles on the integument, which are accompanied by increasing weakness of sensation and loss of voice.

The indolent tubercles characteristic of leprosy show themselves on different parts of the skin; they are hard, uneven, very numerous, grouped closely together, and cause the loss of hair on the spot where they are present. They end in destructive ulceration; these ulcers penetrate to the bones and ultimately produce caries of the bones. Sometimes they lead to the separation of different parts, such as fingers or big toes. To these symptoms are added slowness of movement, obscuration of the senses, alteration of the voice, fœtid breath, mental deterioration.

Three kinds of leprosy are recognized, which have been called squamous, incrusted, and tubercular, according to whether the skin is covered with scales, crusts, or tubercles.

Treatment.—Relatively long and difficult, but result is certain. For a fortnight give S. At the third dilution alt. with the ordinary dose of C. The disease will at first seem much increased, but the patient will soon be reassured by a marked improvement. After this fortnight, external treatment must be added, viz. :—twice a week baths of C^5. G. E. in compresses on the diseased parts.

Warts (Condylomata Excrescences.)

(*See* Tumours.)

DISORDERS OF THE EXTREMITIES, AND CASUALTIES.

Hand (Weakness of).

Contraction, the result of wounding a nerve.

Treatment.—S. in dilution. Compresses to the nerves of the hand of W. E. alt. B. E., or R. E. alt. Y. E. Baths of C5. Compresses of W. E.

Coxalgia.

Affections of the Coxo-femoral articulation—or hip joint—presenting all the anatomical and physiological characteristics of white swelling in the joints.

In the first stage Coxalgia only shows itself by dull and deep pain in the hip. At first intermittent and uncertain, this pain becomes fixed and more acute; very often it is more felt at the knee than at the hip itself.

In *the second stage* the limb is lengthened: in the third stage it is shortened: and those two follow as cause and effect.

In fact, the elongation of the limb is the consequence of change in the articular surfaces and thickening of them. But when this change has as so far advanced that the cotyloid cavity is no longer deep enough to lodge and hold in its place the head of the femur, this bone is dragged out of its socket by the muscles attached to it, and then the ordinary symptoms of dislocation are produced. In fact, the structural changes of the affected parts follow the course which is natural to them; abscesses are formed in and around the joint, and in the majority of cases the patient succumbs to disease. For spontaneous Coxalgia does not consist in a simple local lesion, but is always connected with general constitutional disorder, usually of a scrofulous character. Accordingly in the treatment of this disease the cause must be taken into account, and in most cases, especially if taken under treatment early enough, it can be easily overcome by our Electro-Homœopathic remedies.

Treatment.—If the patient is lymphatic, dil. L. or S. should be given, and application of R. E. to the end of the femur, and to the superficial nerves of the leg—night and morning. If the lymphatic state is very marked, give S. alt. C., and if the constitution is mixed, S. alt. A., 1 globule of C^5. dry every half-hour; and in obstinate cases, C^5., and A^2. alternately, dry. Baths of C^5. or of S^5. alt. L. Compresses over the femur of W. E. Compresses and unctions of C^5.

In spontaneous Coxalgia the treatment is of longer duration, but a cure can be obtained.

Cutting Wounds.

Cuts in the flesh, with loss of blood.

Treatment.—Wash with water containing A. (20 globules to the glass); the flow of blood will be checked at once. Compresses of B. E. may be added, covered in by larger compresses soaked with a lotion of A^2. (20 globules to the glass). These compresses, constantly renewed, have even healed arteries in very severe cases.

Sprains

Resulting from a violent strain of the soft parts surrounding the joints.

Treatment.—S. in dilution. Repeated compresses of R. E. or G. E.

Dislocations

Must be treated according to the constitutional type.

Treatment.—A. or S. Application of R. E. or B. E. In obstinate cases C. in dilution and baths of C5.

Fractures.

The surgeon must be called in to set a fracture, but internal treatment will hasten cure.

Treatment.—S. in dilution, second dilution. Baths, unctions and compresses of C5., S5., or B. E. Applications of R. E. alt. B. E. to the related nerves.

Burns

Are cured by S. externally, and if severe, by S. dil. internally, and compresses of W. E.

When a burn has taken place a compress of R. E. should be at once applied; or else W. E.: and subsequently, on the top of it, a much larger compress of S. (20 globules to the glass of water).

This has always succeeded when it has been tried. If there is a wound complicating the burn, apply compresses of B. E.

Amputation.

Before and after operation, A3. in dilution; and after the surgical dressing has been applied, sprinkle with lotion of A3., 20 globules dissolved in about 6 oz. of water.

Sciatica.

Sciatica is an excessively violent pain, extending from the fold of the buttocks to the hip, the thigh, down one of the legs. The pain is worse in the evening or night, and after food. It arises from a want of vitality, or of conductivity, or discontinuance of nerve currents in the sciatic nerve: rarely from excess of vital force.

Treatment.—Applications of electricity almost always remove the pain. We must begin with R. E., applying it to the one point out of the three, which may be taken in the course of the sciatic nerve, where the pain is most severe. Usually this is the upper point. If R. E. is not sufficient, it must be alternated with Y. E.

Very severe sciatic pain has been entirely removed by the hypo-dermic injection of W. E.

In the rare cases in which the electricities do not act we must have recourse to unctions of C^5. and A^2. to the same nerve points. In all cases the electricities must be used as adjuvantia to the internal treatment. The remedy required is almost always S. or S. alt. C. second dilution.

For angioitic temperaments R. E. and Y. E. must be replaced by B. E. Add A. dil. and baths, unctions and compresses of A^2. Compresses of A^2. over the heart.

Sciatica may be complicated with biliary calculus, which is then the chief cause of suffering. In this case the *treatment* is dil. F. second dilution. Unctions and compresses of F^2. or C^5. to the hypochondria. Application of R. E., alt. Y. E. to the three sciatic points; also to the solar plexus, the sympathetic and the renal regions. Compresses of W. E. to the same points. Baths of C^5.

Legs.

Tumour or soft œdema, painless, often arising from some disorder in the region of the heart.

Treatment.—A^2. in dilution, or C., second dilution. Baths of C^5. alt. A^2. Compresses and unctions of A^2. Unctions of F^2. to the hypochondria. Application of the B. E. to the occiput, sympathetic, and all the nerves of the leg.

Varicose Ulcer.

The same treatment, and compresses of A^2. alt. C^5. (20 globules to a glass of water).

KNEE.

White swelling of the knee.

Treatment.—S. in dilution alt. C. Baths of C^5. Application of R. E., alt. Y. E. to the related nerves. Unctions and compresses of C^5. When there is pain, application of G. E. Unctions of C^5. Compresses of W. E. or B. E.

PERIODICAL RHEUMATISM IN THE KNEE.

Treatment.—F. in dilution, second dilution. Unctions of F^2. to the hypochondria. The treatment is similar to that of gout.

FEET.

Excessive foot-sweat.

Treatment.—Dil. S. alt. A. first dilution. The same remedies, dry. 5 globules of each once daily. Baths of C^5., or S., or A^3., or W. E.

CORNS,

Or callosities, or bunions on the feet.

Treatment.—Dil. S. Unctions of S., 20 globules to the ounce of Cerate. C^5. in unctions also is very successful.

DROWNING.

Treatment.—8 or 10 globules on the tongue, repeated as often as necessary; then as soon as the patient has recovered consciousness, S. in dilution in the first dilution. Application of R. E. alt. Y. E. to the grand sympathetic, solar plexus, and occiput; at first the external remedies must be applied frequently, till some amount of recovery has been attained.

WOUNDS, CONTUSIONS, INJURIES, LACERATIONS, BRUISES.

To allay pain, if there is no hæmorrhage, apply W. E. or G. E.

If there is hæmorrhage, compresses of A. (15 or 20 globules to the glass); if necessary, dil. A., second dilution. Compresses of W. E. or of B. E. act with certainty.

If there is a threatening of gangrene, give dil. C., second dilution, or C. alt. S.

S. causes prompt cicatrization of wounds; and if the wound is due to shock, that is, a sort of contusion of the blood vessels, give A.

Contusions.

"Black and blue" injuries (Ecchymosis), consequent upon falls or blows upon the head or elsewhere.

Treatment.—At the time, compresses of R. E. or B. E., covered in by larger compresses of S. (15 or 25 globules to the glass). When bleeding is stopped compresses of W. E. and S.

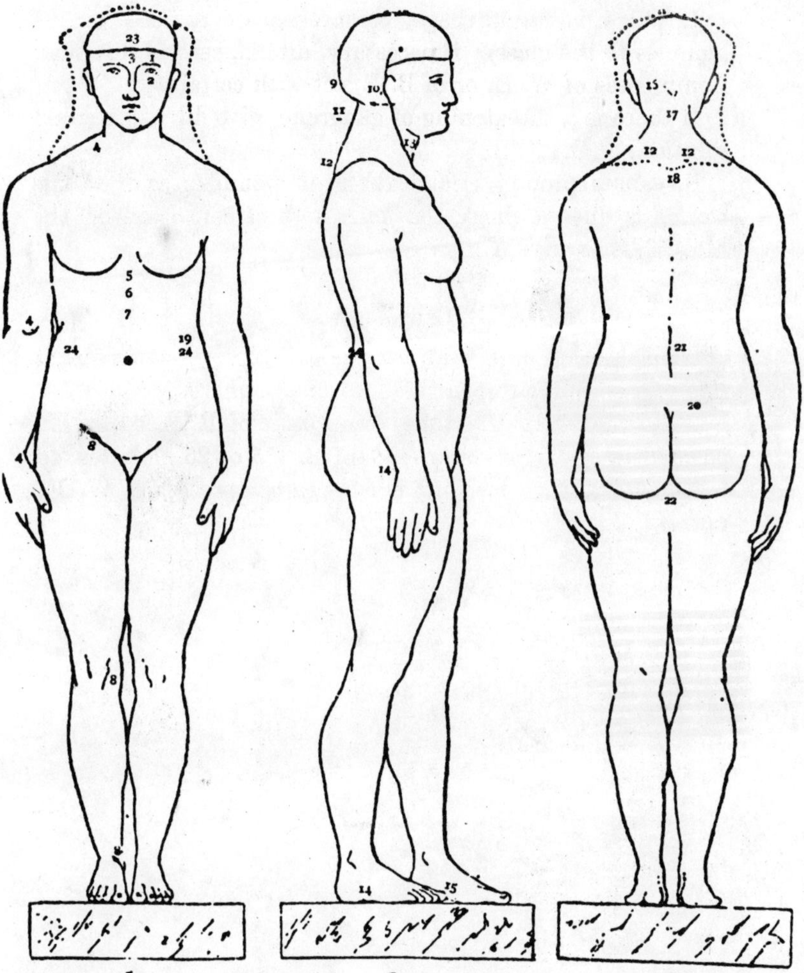

1 2 3

1. Super-orbital.
2. Sub-orbital.
3. Base of nose.
4. Brachial.
5. Solar-Plexus.
6. Pit of Stomach.
7. Gastric Sympathetic.
8. Crural.
9. Little hypoglossi.
10. Little muscles behind the ear.
11. Occiput.
12. Sympathetic.
13. Great hypoglossi.
14. Sciatic nerve.
15. Arch of the Foot.
16. Little hypoglossi.
17. Occiput.
18. Sympathetic (7th vertebræ).
19. Bottom of stomach.
20. Sacral nerves corresponding to parts.
21. Loins.
22. Perineum.
23. Forehead.
24. Hypochondria.

APPENDIX.

Extract from the "Revue Française d'Electro-Homœopathie," August, 1883. By Dr. Labonnardière.

In spite of the example set to us by most of our colleagues, directors and editors of Reviews, or of scientific popular and medical journals, addressed both to men of the world and to independent and progressive physicians, we disclaim in these pages any political bias, or polemic aim, or medical, industrial, or commercial prepossessions. For we know that in all subjects there are adversaries, and these probably form the majority, who are not to be convinced except by the logic of facts, which are of all arguments the hardest and the most invincible; or by the concurrence of time, which often promotes yesterday's absurdity or to-day's paradox into to-morrow's verity,—by the resistless gravitation, in a word, of general common sense, which may be sometimes confused or dazzled by some notion which has the vantage of present possession, or which may be bewildered and overshadowed by some failure of judgment, yet in due time recovers itself. All those who oppose themselves to fact, to time, to common sense, must yield; for, in the progress of truth, the fatal words *too late* can never present an invincible barrier, can never bury truth in the irrecoverable past.

Every medical reality, whatever it refers to, belongs of right to us. We think it therefore our duty to-day to present to our readers a narrative of that terrible malady which becomes in our time increasingly prevalent, under the influence of depressing occupations and overwhelming passions, and which has stricken with its fatal dart the last descendant of the elder branch of the children of Henry IV., the inheritor of the honours of the Bourbon race, and of a royalty of fourteen centuries. His memory is henceforth enshrined in the sentiment of Europe and of the world.

The Comte de Chambord has just succumbed, after an illness lasting several months, apparently from a chronic disease apparently of only a few months' duration, although dating probably from several years. For its roots must be found in the bitterness of exile, in the patriotic laments awakened by the disasters of his country, the cruel disappointments, in fine, which have resulted in the shattering of all the hopes which seemed to promise an early fruition. In plain words, he has died from cancer of the stomach, according to the first diagnosis which was published, and which we believe to be the truest. The published results of a more formal *post-mortem* investigation pronounce the case to have been one of ulceration of the stomach, with or without tumour, complicated with injury to the æsophagus, atrophy of the kidneys, aneurism of the aorta, and other grave organic diseases.

At the beginning of July the disease from which the prince was suffering was announced only by the *Union* journal. Other journals, well informed no doubt, but less judicious, spoke of it earlier—in the middle of May. The first publication of this information startled the public mind like a thunder-bolt, and rumours and suspicions of criminal poisoning were not wanting in the bewilderment and emotion inevitably arising from such a calamity when it was first known. These, of course, were contradicted in the most authentic way; which, indeed, was scarcely necessary in point of the scientific absurdity of the idea that a toxic cause of this kind could produce such a gradual decline of vital force. The medical world could not long remain ignorant of the real nature of the case.

All the reserve, all the designed sophistications of doctors and surgeons of the highest rank, both French and foreign, who were summoned to give the aid which their light and zeal could supply, could not alter the impression which well-informed medical men necessarily formed as they followed the bulletins, with all their significant details, which day after day issued from Frohsdorff. And yet, at the first, we were constrained to suspend judgment at the earlier stages, when we had no guide but the partial and purposely obscure reports to guide us. Judging from a distance, we could not tell whether the diagnosis should be acute gastritis or gouty disease of the stomach taking a rapid course, with advancing ulceration of the gastric mucous membrane; or cancer of the stomach, undetected at first, insidious in its march, moving on more or less slowly. But, in any case, the too probable prognosis made us apprehend inevitable death from inanition.

However, the daily and consecutive indications of destructive cancerous disease, the vomiting of glairy substances, then of food, the alternate relief and exacerbation, the frequent relapses, and then subsequent changes for the better, especially under the influence of a liquid diet rigorously maintained,—the concurrent rapid emaciation, the absolute prostration of strength, the characteristic pallor, the wasting to a skeleton, which the daily papers reported as the unequivocal condition of the august patient,—these signs were not to be mistaken by those who knew the distinctive features of the disease. Lastly, the intolerable sufferings, agonizing and indescribable, of the last fortnight, all the more distressing because, as is usual in such cases, the patient retained to the last, with the exception of transient lapses, the most complete command of his faculties, a perfectly lucid intelligence, normal emotional and voluntary power, while suffering the pangs of slow starvation—this group of symptoms gave increasing probability to the diagnosis which was from the first pronounced by the celebrated Vienna physicians, Drs. Mayr, Diasche, and Billroth. Their conjectures were confirmed by the autopsy, which took place on the 26th of August, in the presence of our illustrious Professor Vulpain, by Drs. Drasche and Mayr, the acting physicians, and Dr. Stanzl, deputed to be present by the authorities of Newstadt.

Thus the diagnosis and prognosis which were made at the outset, when Professor Vulpain was associated in the consultation which took place on the 15th and 16th of July, were verified by the fatal termination of the disease and *post-mortem* demonstration. Nevertheless, the case being that of one of the most constitutionally vigorous men, in the plenitude of strength and health but a little time previously, with a rare capability, judging by the standard generally met with, of vital resistance,—attacked by a disease, which for two or three months indicated its presence by gastric disturbance which he himself treated lightly, the potentates of medical art were enforced at once to pronounce a verdict of condemnation, without the possibility of reprieve. We are indeed convinced that they did all that their knowledge and their conscientious zeal could dictate or suggest to save a patient on whom the gaze of the world was concentrated. And yet they were obliged to confess themselves helpless, or rather that their art was powerless, and to limit themselves to expectant treatment, fortified by the well-known precepts of hygiene, an alimentary regime appropriate to the enfeebled stomach. Soon they were obliged to trust almost entirely to injections of morphia as a last resort, an evil often worse than the disease, in order to suppress the poignant anguish of the cancerous disease. Truly here medicine is seen in despair. May we not, in the presence of such a case, cry out with Claude Bernard—"Surely the therapeutic art is not yet born, and never will be."

Might they have done otherwise? Could a more hopeful course have been suggested? This is the question which naturally arises in every mind who has thoroughly investigated, copiously tested, and intelligently appreciated, with perceptions medically educated, the new medical system of Count Mattei. Its brilliant successes, as well as its occasional more or less partial failures, in the treatment of such diseases as those which were demonstrated to exist in the case of the Count de Chambord, all force this question to the front. With all possible diffidence, with unfeigned respect for the memory of a prince who could win such devotion as that which was freely accorded to him, and for the distinguished physicians whose character and accomplishments we honour and admire—still the question forces itself,—Could nothing more have been done?

We must, of course, admit there is a Providence which determines these events; and that this Supreme Control would not grant a miracle in answer to the many faithful prayers. But might it not have given another triumph to a therapeutic method which has been observed by a large number of distinguished physicians for twenty-five years, both in the hands of Count Mattei, its illustrious discoverer, at Bologna, at Rome, at Rochetta. The doctors themselves, and many persons without any knowledge of medicine, have secured triumphant results, have wrought marvellous achievements in a great number of cases of desperate disease,—cancerous and arthritic disorders of all kinds and of all degrees of severity. Might not such a therapeutic method, we say, win an absolute and decisive victory over the regnant science, which can neither recognize nor admit any innovations outside the enclosures of its schools and academies.

Among the innumerable remedies which were sent from all

parts of the world, among the suggestions addressed from all sides, if we may believe the information and the rumours that circulated during the last two months of that illustrious life, to the different physicians who were summoned to Frohsdorff, were the remedies of Count Mattei sent?—was there any suggestion that the august patient should be treated by Electro-Homœopathy?

Perhaps so. And there is less reason to wonder at this when we know that in more than one European Court the Count Mattei counts princes and even rulers among his clients. May we not, however, affirm that some hope might have been derived from this treatment, which was not resorted to, whether or not it was suggested to his physicians or attendants, in the cure of a disease which, like a slow poison, introduced into the blood by the pining nostalgia of an expatriated citizen and a dethroned monarch, had for a long time extended its ravages through the entire organism.

No one can venture to assert this positively, although there are cases of cancer in the stomach, even at an advanced stage in their development, which have been radically and permanently cured by Electro-Homœopathy. These have been repeatedly attested in various books or publications relating to the new medicine which have appeared during the last twenty-five years. Even if a complete cure could not have been effected, it does not appear doubtful that the wise and timely intervention of Electro-homœopathic treatment, when the earlier dyspeptic manifestations of disease presented themselves, especially the vomiting, which would at once have suggested to an experienced practitioner the possibility of cancerous disease in the digestive system, might have given some favourable chances of uprooting the disease, and of confronting step by step its continued development and extension to neighbouring organs. Its fatal progress might have been retarded by methods adapted to promote nutrition; or, at any rate, so precious a life might have been prolonged, and the excruciating sufferings, which, as we have seen, exist in the great majority of cases of internal cancer, might have been assuaged, and almost completely suppressed.

We might hesitate in dwelling so strongly on these considerations, which we might support by the recital of a great number of cases occurring under our own personal observation, before and since adopting the methods and remedies of Count Mattei in cancerous cases. But we consider, once for all, that we should not be discharging the duty which we owe to our own conscience, if we did not deduce the lessons and counsels which this case suggests, and which are so likely to be profitable to those who favour us with their confidence. These must now rally round the medical system which acts and resists disease—the system which has been already tested, but may yet advance to a higher level of progress,—which has already cured, and is still curing, numberless patients, whose cases are from the first looked upon as hopeless. This method alone has the power of following disease into the deepest recesses of the human organism; and, if that organism is fatally attacked, yet it can at least assuage and minimize the most frightful sufferings that can test human endurance. Help thyself, and heaven will assist thee.

INSTRUCTIVE CASES CURED.

Abscess.—A woman aged 28 years. Abscess on the thigh. Operation unsuccessful; fever. Was cured in eleven days by F^2 alt. S^2. Externally: Compresses of A^2. Unctions of S.

Abscess.—A young woman aged 16. Scrofulous abscess in the ankle joints: stoppage of menstruation; incapable of work. Cured in four weeks by S^2 internally. Unctions of S. Compresses of A^2.

Abscess in the leg; almost paralysed. Cured by S. in dil. Unctions of S. Application of R. E. to the related nerves.

Abscess.—A poor woman, suffering from two abscesses in the arms, caused by the rupture of a tendon. Could not move the arm; had lasted two months. She was completely cured by C. internally. Unctions and compresses of C^4.

Abscess.—Child, 11 years old, suffering from a very red, inflamed abscess at the elbow. All the ointments and incisions employed had not succeeded in reducing or relieving it. 10 globules of L. dry on the tongue, and compresses of L., caused the abscess to break in twenty-four hours. Complete and rapid cure by the internal and external use of L.

Abdomen.—Inflammation of the pancreas.—B. M., aged 40, cured by S. in dil. alt. F. second dilution. Application of R. E. to the sympathetic and the solar plexus.

Abdomen.—Inflammation of the peritonœum after confinement. J., aged 24. F., first glass, rapidly reduced the fever. Cure by C. in dil., and twenty globules dry of the same medicine.

Acne.—Very obstinate case in a girl of 18, had lasted four or five years. The face was entirely covered, the skin livid, and so painful as often to provoke weeping. A^2 and C^3, with occasional use of F^1; unctions of S^5 and baths of C^5 dispersed the eruption in a few months. The cure was lasting.

Anasarca.—One of the most remarkable cases of cure recorded, effected by our medicines, is certainly that of a lady aged 30, living in Brittany.

This lady was attacked by soft œdema or anasarca, a dropsical swelling and infiltration in both legs, caused by heart disease, and an extremely rheumatic and lymphatic constitutional type. The œdema had so far advanced as not only to produce deformity in the feet, but even to soften the bones, so that the poor lady could not walk. As soon as she attempted to support herself on her legs it seemed to her that they were leaden. This disease had continued for some years and was continually increasing. For more than a year the legs had been swollen, and for several months the patient had been confined to her bed or her couch.

After having tried, without result, all the treatment which could be suggested by the doctors of her own town and the neighbourhood, the patient was removed to Paris, in order to consult there the most distinguished physicians. At Paris, as in Brittany, the case was pronounced to be complicated by softening of the bones, and the doctors did not disguise their impressions of the extreme gravity of the case.

Under these circumstances she decided to resort to Electro-Homœopathy. The principal remedies used were dilutions of A. and of S. internally; compresses of A^3 over the heart; compresses of S. and of C^5 on the legs and feet; and immersion baths of S. and C^5.

During the first weeks of treatment, a perceptible improvement manifested itself in her general state, and in less than three months she was able to consider herself entirely cured. From that time she resumed her ordinary habits, her strength returned and increased daily.

Anœmia.—G. E. was suffering from anœmia, had been

ordered by her doctors to keep her bed for a month, as she could not walk, and could scarcely take any food. All stimulants and tonics were interdicted, under the pretext that she was too weak to take them. She was cured in forty days by A. internally, and A. and S. externally.

Aneurism of the Aorta.—Mr. E. P., aged 38, suffered from aortic aneurism. After three months treatment by A., first dilution, and light applications of B. E. over the heart, he was completely cured.

Angina.—Mrs. L. P., aged 28, was cured in three days of angina, with high fever, so violent in character that typhoid fever was apprehended, by C^5 in dil, and unctions of F^2 to the hypochondria.

Angioitis, or general vascular congestion.—Mr. L. F., aged 40, was threatened with paralysis from general plethora. In two months he was entirely cured by A. internally and externally, and the use of B. E.

A similar case in the Baroness A. was cured in a few days by the internal use of A.

Anchylosis.—T. P., aged 58, had had anchylosis for a year; she was entirely cured in three months by S. internally and the external application of W. E.

Aphonia.—Miss A. J., aged 19, had suffered loss of voice for eighteen months; all allopathic remedies had been used. She was directed to take P. alt. S., in the second glass. Compresses and unctions of S. to the throat. Under this treatment an eruption appeared over the whole body, but the chest was considerably relieved. A. was substituted for S. Sixteen days afterwards a violent fit of coughing brought a clot of black blood into the mouth; then, by a most natural coincidence, the pain at the apex of the lungs entirely disappeared. The previously-existing pain had apparently been caused solely by this little deposition of blood, which had dispersed under the action of A. The voice gradually returned, and in a month it was completely restored.

Aphonia.—Miss V., aged 16, had completely lost her voice in consequence of a chill. For six days it was impossible to understand her when she attempted to speak. She was cured in half an hour by the application of R. E. to the hypoglossi, the occiput, the great sympathetic, the solar plexus, and especially to the pit of the stomach, and by washing the throat with S. lotion, twenty globules to the tumblerful.

Apoplexy.—Cured in three months by A. internally, and B. E. externally.

Arthritis.—Mr. S. D., aged 42. Was suffering from very severe arthritis; he was cured in one month by S. in the first dilution, and the use of R. E. alternately with Y. E. to the joints affected.

Arthritis.—Mr. C. C., aged 58. Suffering from chronic arthritis. Was cured in two months by S. internally.

Arthritis.—Arthritic inflammation of the first joint of the index finger, and erysipelas of the dorsum of the hand. Was cured in three months by S. internally, and unctions of A^2.

Arthritis.—Of five years' standing. Was cured by the alternate application of R. E. alt. Y. E.; immersion baths of C^3 and dilution of S.

Arthritis.—Another chronic case of five years' standing. The joints recovered movement after internal cure had been effected by A., and one drop of W. E. daily in a spoonful of water, and alternate applications of R. E. and Y. E.

Asphyxia.—O. P., aged 16, seized with asphyxia from inhalation of carbonic acid gas, with convulsions. Was cured in a month by A. internally, and W. E. externally, applied to the centre of the skull.

Asthma.—Nervous asthma for twenty-five years. P. S., aged 56. Was cured in six months by S., second dilution, and application of R. E. to the great sympathetic, the solar plexus, the occiput, and the pit of the stomach.

Asthma.—Mr. L., aged 68, suffering from asthma for six years, consequent on frequently recurring bronchitis, and tendency to catarrh. The disease had resisted all treatment, even change of climate. In three weeks a notable improvement was produced by A. alternately with S. in the first dilution, and P^3, second dilution. Application of R. E. to the great sympathetic, the solar plexus, and occiput. Unctions on the chest of C^4. In two months the cure was complete.

Atrophy.—S. J., a child of 2 years. A characteristic type of scrofulous atrophy; was cured and entirely transformed in a few weeks by A. alternately with C., and the application of R. E.

WOUNDS.—Z. G., aged 22. When hunting, his gun burst, and was wounded in the radius, near the right wrist; he had a scrofulous constitution. Was cured by S. internally. Application of R. E. alt. Y. E. Unctions of A. alt. C.

WOUND.—A gun-shot accident to the tendon achilles (heel). Stiffness of the foot, which was pronounced incurable, threatening of gangrene. Pains were subdued by R. E., and he was cured by C.

WOUND.—A woman had been struck on the face by a bar of iron. The bone was smashed, the cheek lacerated, the face swollen, great loss of blood and extreme pain. B. E. and compresses of A. arrested bleeding; and W. E. alt. G. E. quickly removed the pains and reduced the swelling.

STOMATITIS.—Mr. O. S. was suffering from chronic syphilitic inflammation in the mouth; was cured in two months by the following treatment. S. alt. with Ven. in dilution. Gargles of C. alt. with S. Application of R. E. alt. Y. E. to the pit of the stomach.

BRONCHITIS.—A man aged 36 had chronic bronchitis and indigestion; of a mixed temperament. Cured by P., in the second dilution, and S. taken at meals.

BRONCHITIS.—Mrs. H. M. had been suffering for nearly four months from bronchitis, when she resolved to try Electro-Homœopathy. By taking P. she was cured in five weeks.

BRONCHITIS.—Mrs. X., aged 67, suffering from bronchitis and hæmorrhage. Was cured by A. in dilution, alternately with P.; and by L. alternately with S., taken in wine at meals.

BRONCHITIS AND ERYSIPELAS.—A. K., aged 24, single, was seized by bronchitis and violent erysipelas. Alarming state, constant delirium, pulse 136, temperature 104°, tongue perfectly dry. Weakness was so great that the patient could not expectorate the mucus secreted. Erysipelas on the left side extended from the back as far as the thigh, and from the left hand up to the elbow. S. alt. A. alt. P., third dilution. Compresses of A^2 on the erysipelatous parts. Unctions of F^2 to the hypochondria. After twenty-four hours the disease had entirely changed in appearance; in six days the erysipelas and all dangerous symptoms had disappeared. In a week the case was completely cured.

CHRONIC BRONCHITIS.—A man, aged 48, suffering from chronic bronchitis and hæmorrhage from the lungs at every change of season, spring and autumn. He was treated in 1880 with A. alternately with P., and an eruption appeared all over the whole body. He then found a general improvement of health and strength returned. This treatment was continued for some time, and the cure was complete, for during three years subsequently, there has been no return of the attack.

Chronic Bronchitis.—A man, aged 58, had suffered for two years from bronchitis and constant cough. Expectoration viscid and greenish; night perspirations; much oppression of breath, hindering movement; emaciation. Cured by P., A., and C.

Burn.—A child of 3; severe burns in the hands. Quickly cured by lotions of L., 20 globules to the glass.

Calculus.—In the kidneys. A woman suffering from leucorrhœa and general debility. Took C. alternately with S., second dilution. After eight hours the leucorrhœa had diminished, sleep and appetite returned. After a fortnight's treatment she passed from the kidneys a quantity of red sand mixed with white round scales about one-sixth of an inch in diameter, and many others of different shapes, but smaller. She was completely cured.

Calculus.—A man of 55, very powerful; had been treated allopathically for stone for some time. Cured by S. alternately with A. internally; baths and compresses of S. and of W. E.

Cancer.—Open cancer of the breast. Madame Gualdi, of Rome, had a cancer extending to under the arms, with caries of the ribs; pronounced incurable; the right arm swollen, incapable of movement; muscles of the neck drawn, and the head bent towards the shoulder. The case was treated by Professor Pascucci, from April 4, 1869, to June 6, 1870. Cure completed by C.

Cancer.—In the breast. Albina Masotti, having passed eight years in different hospitals, and been sent home to die, was cured in one year, and lived in Bologna for several years.

Cancer.—In the nose. Tonioli Pietro, aged 64. Nose destroyed; after four months treatment by C. was cured, and the nose was restored by plastic operation.

Cancer.—Madame Zanotti Rosa, aged 44, cancer in the right axilla (arm-pit) of four years' standing; cured in eleven months by C. The patient is still living at Poggio Renatico.

Cancer.—Madame Zoboli Maddalena, aged 47 years; cured by C. of uterine cancer, after unsuccessful allopathic treatment.

Madame Grazia Maria, aged 48; cured of uterine cancer by C. C^5.

Madame Marguerite Bagnoli, aged 54; cured of uterine cancer by C.

CANCER.—On the tongue, extending beyond; cured by C^2. Mr. Pellago Crispino, aged 48.

CANCER.—On the thigh. Mr. Gaetano Lindri, aged 59; cured ten years ago by C., and is still living at Bologna (Borgo dell' Ora, No. 496).

CANCER.—A woman, at the critical age, was attacked by inflammation of the nose and lips, during five months she was subjected to allopathic treatment; but her state became steadily worse. The doctor was obliged to inform the relatives of the patient that he regarded it as carcinoma, and that cure was impossible.

She then resolved to employ the Electro-Homœopathic remedies, and the patient took A. alternately with C. internally, and compresses of A^2 on the nose and lips. She also applied B. E. to the root of the nose. In two months she was cured.

PALPITATIONS AND CONVULSIONS.—A little girl of 12; was treated for these diseases by A., second glass; and unctions of A^2 over the heart. A few days afterwards she had a convulsive attack, and then remained quite well. But being also troubled with liver disorder, she took F. alternately with A. After two months she was completely cured, and was able to go to work in the factory, where she is still employed.

CANCEROUS PHARYNGITIS.—Mr. Jaetano Pura, aged 32; cured by C.; is still living at Caselle, Bologna.

ULCERATION OF THE UTERUS.—Madame Carolina Cherubina, aged 19; cured by C.

ULCER OF PYLORUS.—Mr. Sante Masini, aged 62; cured by C.

CANCEROUS ULCERATION OF THE RIGHT LEG, consequent upon wound and fracture of the tibia. Del Rosso, soldier; cured by C.; still living.

UTERINE POLYPUS.—Treated for three years allopathically, without result, and pronounced incurable. Madame Angela Cuppini; cured by C. nine years ago, and is still living.

SCIRRHUS OF THE BREAST.—Madame Geltrude Baldi, aged 54; cured by C.

Similar case: Madame Caterini Mazzetti; cured by C; still living.

SCIRRHUS OF THE BREAST.—Madame Cecilia Monte; cured by C.

SCIRRHUS OF THE RIGHT BREAST.—Treated by several physicians without result, and pronounced incurable. Madame Nanni Rosa, aged 45; cured twelve years ago by C.; is still living in perfect health.

SCIRRHUS OF THE BREAST.—Madame Anna Pancald, aged 52; cured by C.

SCIRRHUS OF THE BREAST.—Madame Candida Finelli, aged 61; cured by C.

SCIRRHUS OF THE BREAST.—The Duchess Ravarchieri Freschi, shortly after the death of her mother, Princess Filangeri, who had died at Naples of cancer, came to Bologna to be operated upon by a celebrated surgeon. Under the action of C., without any operation, the Duchess was perfectly cured, and after ten years she is still living in the enjoyment of good health.

SCIRRHUS OF THE RIGHT BREAST.—Anna Venturi, of Calvenzano, province of Bologna, aged 46, widow of Paul Mattioli, *propriétairê*, was attacked by scirrhus in the right breast. She was under the treatment of the local doctor, and was sent to Bologna to be operated upon by the learned Professor Boretti, in November, 1876. The operation was ably performed, the whole mass removed, and the surgeon assured her that it would not return. But in February, 1877, the scirrhus did return, in the same breast. Again she put herself under the care of her medical attendant, and he advised her to submit herself to a second operation; accordingly, she once more visited Bologna to be operated upon by M. Loretta. A third time, also, operation was performed by Professor Massarenti, since, in April, 1878, the scirrhus reappeared, as if it had never been removed. Still the scirrhus tumour, although so resolutely confronted, proved irrepressible, and presented itself a fourth time, but in another form, in the form of an enormous wound on the left leg. At last, in desperation, she determined to test the resources of Rochetta, and in sixty-three days—in nine weeks—by means only of C., used internally and externally, she was perfectly cured, and remains so, as any one may ascertain, by making inquiries at Calvenzano.

SCIRRHUS OF THE STOMACH.—Mr. Domenico Arioni, aged 32; cured by C

Two Scirrhus Tumours of the Stomach.—Monsignor Grent, Bishop of Sutwart, came to Rome, wasted, a wreck, with two scirrhus tumours in his stomach; he could not keep anything on his stomach, even water or broth. In one month he was able to eat like a healthy man. But his character was so active that he overworked himself, and at the same time interrupted treatment; a fatal relapse followed.

Uterine Scirrhus; advancing rapidly and not to be controlled. Diagnosed by the celebrated Professor Rizzoli.—Melazzi Assunta was cured in a month by C., eleven years ago; she is still living, and well, at Bologna.

Uterine Scirrhus: treated without result for four years by Dr. Tinti.—Madame Maria Gavazini was treated fourteen years ago, and cured by C., and is still living at Vigorso.

Uterine Scirrhus.—Madame Laurea Palmieri, aged 55; cured by C.

Uterine Scirrhus.—Campionesi, a widow, aged 55; cured by C., and is still living.

Uterine Scirrhus.—Madame Tabellini Teresa, of Bologna; pronounced incurable by several physicians; cured, and still living.

Uterine Scirrhus: relapse after operation by Professor Rizzoli, and declared incurable.—Madame Anna Ghedini; cured.

All these cures occurred anterior to the introduction of the homonyms, the varieties of C., and were obtained by the use of C. alone.

Scirrhus of the Lower Lip: relapse after operation by Professor Rizzoli.—Mr. Matteo Buri; cured by C.

Scirrhus of the Lower Lip—Mr. Innocenzio Donati, aged 85; cured by C.

Scirrhus of the Tongue.—Madame Teresa Conti, aged 47; cured by C.

Scirrhus of the Tongue.—Henry Bolelli, aged 7; cured by C.

Scirrhus of the Pylorus.—Countess Chiassi, of Rome; cured in four months, six years ago. Still living, and in the enjoyment of perfect health.

Scirrhus of the Testicle.—Mr. Gengio Balanzoni, aged 54; cured by C.

Cancerous Tumour of the Uterus.—Madame Madalena Bignani, aged 42; cured by C.

Cancerous Tumour of the Anus, accompanied by another of the same character in the abdomen, in a woman of 50. The external tumour was as large as a child's head, was mapped over by varicose vessels, had extremely deep roots, extending to the vagina, and was subject to formidable hæmorrhages. The general health was so severely affected that the doctor declared that it was too late for operation externally, and that the patient could not live more than a few weeks. The pain was excessive. Three years ago treatment commenced with small doses of all the cancerous medicines, assisted by the angioitics in all doses, with dry globules and immersion baths. The regularity and perseverance with which she followed this treatment was truly admirable, but she was nobly recompensed. Pain ceased, the tumour was reduced by three-quarters of its bulk, after having suppurated profusely; also it became less adherent, and showed a tendency to separate. The general health is most satisfactory; the complexion has become ruddy and fresh, the blood is purified; in a word, there is every indication of a rapid progress toward certain recovery. Perhaps it may not be complete, this is possible; but so far the results are gratifying.

Catarrh.—M. L., aged 64, suffering for many years from gastric catarrh, vertigo, irregular action of the heart. Cured in eight months by S. alt. F., first dilution, A., second dilution, 10 globules, dry, of S. daily, unctionsto the hypochondria of F^2 alt. C^5. Applications of B. E. to the region of the heart, and to the nerves of the head.

Catarrh.—A woman, aged 48, suffering from chronic intestinal catarrh, sometimes diarrhœa, sometimes obstruction, frequent bloody or lemon-coloured evacuations; inertia of the digestive organs; was cured by A. alt. S. alt. F. Unctions of F^2. to the hypochondria.

Catarrh.—A gentleman suffering from intestinal catarrh, was cured in a week by C.

Catarrh.—M. B., aged 50, had been suffering for seven years from gastric and intestinal catarrh, congestion of the liver, asthma, with violent action of the right carotid, and rasping bruit, pronounced incurable. Was completely cured in six months by A. alt. F., alt. S., alt. E. Unctions and compresses of A., F^2, C^5.

Catarrh.—A child, fourteen months, suffered from catarrh, consequent upon acute bronchitis, coming on soon after birth.

Cured by S. alt. P^3, given through the nurse, in the first glass.

CATARRH.—A child, three years, treated homœopathically for five months, was cured in twenty days of chronic intestinal cartarrh and bronchitis, by P. alt. C.

ACUTE PULMONARY CATARRH.—A young man, attacked by acute pulmonary catarrh, and in the opinion of the doctor could not live through the day. Was saved, and promptly restored by S. alt. P., second glass.

CATARRH.—R. H., aged 30, was seized by chronic catarrh and tuberculosis. It is to be noted that this was a relapse, and that the patient had been ill for two years. The double disease was entirely subdued by S. dil., alt. A., alt. F^2, alt. P^4; and application of R. E.

CATARRH.—Madame C. M., suffering for a year from catarrh; was cured in a few weeks by P^3 alt. P^4 internally, and application of R. E. to the centre of the skull.

CATARRH.—Madame M. G., aged 29, suffering for two years from gastric catarrh, irregular heart's action, and tumour in the abdomen. She was cured in four months by S. alt. A., alt. F., first dilution, and C., second dilution. Externally: unctions of C^5 on the abdomen and hypochondria; light compresses of A^2 over the heart.

CEREBRAL DISEASE.—Softening of the brain. Case pronounced incurable. A. M., aged 45, of vigorous constitution, was suddenly seized, in consequence of overwork, with congestion of the brain, threatening softening. The following symptoms soon followed: general appearance of hebetude, involving gradually the whole body; feeling of weight in the occiput; cerebral impressions either destroyed or exaggerated. Cured in two months by C. alt. A., second dilution; unctions of C^5 alt. A^2., alt. S.

CHLOROSIS.—A most interesting case. A young girl of 20, suffering from chlorosis, anæmia, scrofula, and disease of the liver. She dragged on for three years, with no heart for anything except devotional exercises. In a short time there was sensible amelioration under the action of A., C., S., and F. alt. Treatment continues, and she is in a fair way towards complete recovery.

CHOLERINE.—A man had been suffering for two hours from

choleraic symptoms, with cramps in the legs. Ten globules of S. stopped the vomiting; the next day there was one diarrhœic evacuation. Convalescence after two days, by the use of S. The cramps in the legs yielded to unctions of G. E.

In a similar case, without cramp, but accompanied by extraordinary exhaustion, the vomiting and diarrhœa ceased immediately after taking 10 globules, dry, of S. After some hours the patient was fit to rise; treatment was continued by S. in dilution, and the alternate application of R. E. and Y. E.

Chorea, or St. Vitus's Dance.—A child of 11, tormented sinces its birth by chorea, could neither speak, nor keep quiet, nor walk. After being treated by S. and A., and electric washes to the head, it was able to walk one or two miles, and to keep fairly still. Cure was completed after four months' treatment.

Chorea, or St. Vitus's Dance.—A man, aged 26, suffering for three weeks, obliged to keep reclining; cured in two days by S., second dilution.

Heart Disease.—Hypertrophy, with herpes and laceration. Mr. L. M. cured himself in three months of hypertrophy of the heart of twenty years' standing, thoroughly diagnosed by the doctors in attendance, by the use of S. alt. A. third dilution. He was cured of a herpes on the left thigh of six years' standing; it disappeared in three days. He was also cured, under the action of the same treatment, with the addition of A. and A^2, of internal muscular laceration, of nine years' continuance, which had left him exposed to severe pain on the least exertion; and he was habitually deaf. This pain completely ceased to reappear after six months of the same treatment, completed by alcoholic frictions of C^5 on the painful part.

Heart Disease.—P. B., aged 18, suffering for two years from extremely grave heart disease. Besides palpitation and irregularity of the heart's action, there was sometimes great swelling of the aorta, and often even swelling of the whole body, especially the left side. Moreover, he was completely deaf in the left ear, on account of a constant whistling noise in it. Complete cure by A., third dilution, in small doses, unctions of A^2 over the heart and aorta; application of W. E. on the skull and on the principal nerves of the ear.

Heart Disease.—Woman, aged 65, suffering from palpitation, vertigo, weakness, caused by catarrhs resulting from chill.

She was cured by A., first glass. Unctions of A^2 on the head.

HEART DISEASE.—Madame N. suffered from oppression, and violent palpitation, with anguish lasting a week, sleepless, without appetite, fighting for breath. Allopathy could do nothing for her, and the attendant physician expected only speedy death. She was completely cured in a week by A. dil., and compresses of the same remedy on the heart.

HEART DISEASE.—A girl of 7 years; continually liable to bloody evacuations, returning constantly for two days. The heart's action is violent; there is stifling and palpitation. A. was given to her in the third dilution. Applications of W. E. Unctions of A^2. Three hours afterwards blood was discharged from the nose in large clots: then the child slept soundly. She woke completely cured.

HEART DISEASE.—Mr. N. V., aged 31, suffered from excessive palpitation. He was cured in forty-five days by A. internally, and light applications of W. A. over the heart.

HEART.—Aneurism of the aorta, of four years' standing, pronounced incurable; cured by A. in the second dilution, and compresses of A^2.

HEART DISEASE.—Aneurism, with great suffocation; speech jerking and as if broken by sobs. The region of the aorta very painful, not even enduring the weight of a light covering; walking almost impossible. Cured by A. internally and externally. After six months the patient could sing at concerts.

HEART DISEASE.—Organic disease of the heart, complicated with dropsy of the chest, of six months' standing. Cured in one month by A., second glass; compresses of A^2. to the heart.

ORGANIC DISEASE OF THE HEART.—A woman, aged 32, was suffering from organic disease of the heart, well defined; and had been given up by her doctors. Swollen, jaundiced, the poor woman was the object of pity to those who witnessed her extreme suffering. Electro-Homœopathy restored her to life and health by very small doses of A. Unctions of A^2 over the heart. Since her recovery she has borne three children.

COLIC.—A man, aged 68, had suffered for twenty-eight years with colic and vertigo. He was cured by the following treatment. Ver., first dilution, produced a slight amelioration for four days; then no effect. I substituted two globules for one; the effect was more sensible than before; the gastric pains lessened, giddiness less frequent, disturbed vision more transient, and no more fainting. After a fortnight's treatment thus carried out, the dose was increased to three globules each glass; in two days the pains disappeared, and the head remained perfectly free. After three weeks, slight weakness was felt in the head, which disappeared immediately on taking a single dose of the same prepared with four globules.

CONTUSIONS.—F. G., aged 65, had, in consequence of a fall, bruises in the face, with ulceration and threatening of gangrene. He was perfectly cured in a fortnight by C. alt. A. internally, with compresses of C^5 and B. E.

CONVULSIONS.—N. M., aged 40, had suffered almost daily for ten years from convulsions. To her astonishment, the convulsions completely disappeared with the first dose of A., and did not return.

CONVULSIONS.—A woman of 62, cured by S.; convulsions returned every summer; they have not returned since treatment.

CONVULSIONS of severe kind, from fright, removed immediately by the application of R. E. to the sympathetic.

HOOPING COUGH.—Two children, brother and sister, attacked by hooping cough, were cured in four days by P. alt. L., second glass.

COXALGIÂ.—E. R., aged 17, had the thigh-bone dislocated through rheumatic disease. The displacement had existed for three months before she presented herself for treatment. She was cured in a few days by S. internally and R. E. externally.

COXALGIÂ.—J. L., aged 62, suffered from dislocation of the thigh-bone (femur), in consequence of a fall. And as he had a constitutional tendency to rickets, he was subjected to the internal action of S. and R. E. to the femur. He was cured in a short time.

COXALGIÂ.—Madame A., aged 55, suffered from dislocation of the left femur, pronounced incurable. She was cured in a month by S. internally, and baths of R. E.

COXALGIÂ.—Madame M. R., aged 40, accidental coxalgiâ, from a fall. Cured in a fortnight by applying W. E. to the end of the femur, and S. in dilution alt. C.

SPONTANEOUS COXALGIÂ.—A child of 4 years, 8 months. Treated by S., second glass, half a glassful daily; afterwards S^5 in the same dilution, and three globules dry, daily, of C^5; and application of R. E. three times a day to the end of the femur. Head wash of W. E. Cured completely in four months, to the great surprise of his physician.

Spontaneous Coxalgiâ.—A woman, aged 33, very lymphatic, had coxalgiâ first at the age of sixteen. After much treatment, even with the actual cautery to the knee, which was treated for white swelling, amputation was recommended. In consequence of long continued pain she could scarcely walk; the foot only supported by the toes, the leg twisted, contracted, and drawn inwards. Compresses of R. E. to the end of the femur and to the nerves of the leg, and S. in dilution, produced amelioration in three weeks. After four months the heel rested on the ground, the knee was reduced, and complete cure seemed approaching. Cure of spontaneous coxalgiâ is always slow, because the whole mass of the blood must be altered, and the capsule of the joint must be emptied of a secretion which has lodged there, pushing out the femur. On the other hand, cure is always easy and prompt when coxalgiâ is due to some external cause.

Crusta Lactea: Scald head.—A child, 5 years old, suffered from scald head, involving the right eye. The abdomen also had patches of scab scattered over its surface. She was perfectly cured by the internal use of S., third dilution.

Scrofulous Eruption. Psoriasis.—*Case.*—The patient, a lady of 55, suffered from a diffused herpetic state, showing itself especially on the arms, the legs, the knees, and the scalp. This was closely connected with dyspepsia, which was more marked in proportion as the skin disorder temporarily subsided. Functions very irregular; alternate diarrhœa and constipation; indications of gravel; febrile state all right. Also this lady suffered from migraine severely since the disappearance of the menses. Lymphatic temperament.

Treatment began August 19th, 1881, by A^3, second dilution, alternately with C., second dilution. S., one globule, dry, night and morning; baths of C^5 and A^2; unctions of A^2.

The first report, received September 19th, was good. Better nights; nervous movements less violent and frequent; the eruption begins to fade. The treatment was continued till October 28th. Then the globules of S., night and morning, were replaced by F., and four globules of S. were given at each meal.

At this time the paroxysms of fever became stronger, the patient complained of stomach pains and of earthy stools, which justified the change.

December 29.—Severe intermittent fever; digestion painful and difficult; intestinal disturbance almost periodically; bad nights; nervous distress. But the eruption has entirely disappeared. These severe symptoms arose from their retrocession.

A^3, second dilution; C., second dilution; F., first dilution; unctions of A. over the heart; baths of F^2, C^5, and A^2.

April 4, 1882.—The eruption has entirely disappeared; strength has returned; the paroxysms of fever sensibly diminished; but the stomach is less easy, digestion is always difficult; there is constant intestinal disturbance, with colic and nausea.

F., L., A^3, second dilution; baths of C^5 and A^2; unctions of F^2 to the hypochondria; L. during meals.

May 15, 1882.—No change. Mouth bitter and clammy. A^3 and F., second dilution; S^2 in the first dilution; L. at meals; F^2 to the hypochondria.

June 12.—Very slight improvement. Fever, though persistent, is no longer periodic or paroxysmal; nervous disorder is less; the mouth is not bitter; motions more regular.

The same treatment, with less doses, is continued.

July 4.—Continued improvement, but fever continues, and is paroxysmal.

September 4.—Fever, intestinal disorder, weight at the stomach, all have almost disappeared; but the eruption has re-appeared in a few patches on the ear and scalp.

S., first dilution; F., first dilution; A^3, third dilution; L. at meals; unctions and pomade of S; baths of S. and L.

October 9.—No more fever or nervous disorder. The disease might be considered cured, but for the constantly recurring scales on the scalp; also she complains of threatened paralysis of the right arm.

S^2 and S^5, second dilution, F., second dilution; L. at meals; A^2 over the heart; R. E. and dressings of C^5 to the threatened arm.

From this time up to April 9, 1883, reports were constantly and increasingly encouraging. The paralysis of the arm has been warded off, and the treatment continued by F., second dilution; S., first dilution; three globules of C^5, dry, four times a day, and three globules of L. every morning. And now, August 28th, the cure is complete.

HERPETIC ERUPTION.—Mr. B. F., aged 55, had been affected since the age of three years with malignant herpes on the face. Treated at first at Bologna, by Professor Gamberini, during four years with vapour baths and arsenical preparations; then by another Professor with a variety of remedies. He was cured by S. and Ven. internally and externally in the brief space of seven weeks.

DIPHTHERIA.—The parish of Lagaro, Bologna, containing six hundred and forty inhabitants, was the scene of an event which is worthy of public record. Eighty-three persons were attacked by diphtheria. Of these, seventy-eight were treated allopathically, and the seventy-eight all died with allopathic ritual, and were buried with allopathic honours. Five of the eighty-three were treated by the minister, Mr. D. Jean Morelli, by the new medical methods of Electro-Homœopathy, and these five were cured. The treatment was very simple. Gargles of S., A3, R. E., or B. E., and, in very bad cases, washes and unctions of the same remedies (one at a time) to the whole of the throat and neck. It might be expected that those in authority who have some responsibility, and are supposed to have some concern for the welfare of the community, might look into the occurrence of a fact of this gravity and seek for its import; but they pass on their way smiling, and with light hearts and impenetrable calmness they go on with their work with such fatal results for the people.

ACUTE HERPES.—Madame P. M. was suffering from an acute attack of herpes, preventing her entirely from using her hands. She was cured by compresses of C5, and by C. in dilution, internally, alternately with A.

SACCHARINE DIABETES.—Mr. P. S., aged 35, suffering from diabetes of five years' standing, was cured in a short time by S., alternately with A3, and for twenty days. Five drops of B. E. in a glassful of water.

DIPHTHERIA.—A little girl, aged 6, was attacked by diphtheria. The uvula, tonsils, palatal arches, and pharynx were red and swollen. There were some brown patches, surrounded by a circle of inflammation, exuding a purulent secretion. By using forceps the back of the throat was washed every ten minutes with a lotion of C^5 (twenty-five globules to the glass of water). Compresses of F^2 to the hypochondria; unctions of A. alt. S. to the throat; and S. in dilution. A complete cure was effected in a few days.

SCROFULOUS ERUPTION.—Mr. P. had consulted many doctors for a venous eruption on the heel. All had pronounced the case incurable; but he was completely cured by C. alt. A., with unctions and baths of C^5.

TEETH.—A gentleman had suffered twenty days with swellings of the left gums, causing horrible spasmodic suffering. There were no decayed teeth. After two applications of R. E. by the "cupping" process, the pain entirely ceased.

A lady, suffering from spasms, arising from a decayed tooth. Pain ceased on the application of R. E., alternately with Y. E., without the aid of a dentist to extract the tooth.

Many cases of neuralgia in the cheeks, caused by decayed teeth, have been cured by the simple use of the electricity.

DIABETES.—A lady of 68, attacked by saccharine diabetes and eczema of a painful character in the feet, legs often swollen and very painful, was cured by L. internally, and five drops of B. E. on a lump of sugar taken daily; unctions of C^5 and application of B. E.

DIARRHŒA.—A young lady, aged 15, was reduced to a skeleton by constant diarrhœa and complete loss of appetite. All treatment, even homœopathic, had entirely failed. In two months she was quite cured by daily use of S. and occasional use of C.

A child, aged 12, had had diarrhœa for a fortnight, and colic after every meal. R. E. to the stomach and the sympathetic, and four globules of S., cured the case in twelve hours.

PAINFUL ABDOMINAL CONGESTION.—A man, aged 68, suffering from sensation of internal heat, loss of appetite, and spinal pain, treated unsuccessfully by allopathy, was cured in a few days by F., alternately with A. in the second dilution, and unctions of C^5 to the dorsal spine.

DYSPEPSIA.—A lady, aged 52, was cured of dyspepsia and rheumatism in three days by S. internally, and compresses of S^5 and R. E.

NERVOUS DYSENTERY.—A titled lady, aged 63, had been afflicted, since 1881, with dysentery. I saw her on the evening of April 8th, and during the preceding twenty-four hours she had had thirty-four evacuations of white mucus. Each action was attended by frightful griping pains, sometimes extorting cries of distress. I dissolved one globule of S. in about a quart of water, and gave her a teaspoonful every ten minutes. The next day, at nine o'clock, she was much better, and without fever. She had had only five actions during the night. I gave one globule of S. in about a pint of water; and, on the 10th of April, S. in first dilution. On the 11th of April she was completely cured. (*Reported by Dr. Held.*)

DYSMENORRHŒA.—Miss H., aged 18, suffered from very great pain at each return of the monthly illness, pain being in the lower part of the stomach and the sacrum; face very flushed, with palpitation and irregular action of the heart. She was cured in four months by A. alt. C., alt. S., first dilution; unctions, compresses, and baths of A., alternately with C. and S.; application of W. E. to the region of the heart, to the abdomen, and sacrum.

Princess G., aged 20, was seized with severe pains in the same regions, and cured by the same treatment.

Many cases of dysmenorrhœa and amenorrhœa in married and unmarried women have been cured by this same treatment.

EPILEPSY. 1.—Mr. C. C., aged 18, had daily attacks of epilepsy. He was cured in a few days by S., second dilution, A., first dilution, five globules of Ver., dry, at bedtime, and unctions of A^2 over the heart.

2.—Mr. C., aged 47, had had epilepsy for six years. He was cured by S., second dilution, in a few weeks.

3.—Madame L. O., since the age of 16, had had daily attacks of epilepsy. She was quite cured by A., alternately with C., second dilution, and light compresses of A. over the heart.

4.—A child of eight years was attacked by epilepsy, the paroxysms increasing in frequency. The parents first noticed the attack when the child was two years old. It was dosed with bromides, iodides, &c., without result. Electro-Homœopathic treatment began with S. in the first dilution, and the attacks became more frequent. Then the third dilution of S. was at once given; the attacks became weaker and less frequent, but did not cease. Having observed that the child often picked at its nose, the treatment was modified as follows:—S^3 alternately with Ver., third dilution; a teaspoonful every two hours. For ten days no observable result was produced; the state remained unchanged. But on the eleventh day colic set in, with putrid motions, and the epileptic attacks at once became milder and less frequent. The treatment was continued. After a month the remedies were given in the first dilution, and the last paroxysm occurred thirteen months after the commencement of treatment. In thirty-one months the child became very lively and intelligent. It may be supposed that the attacks were not primarily epileptic, but were caused by the presence of worms.

5.—L. Z., woman aged 39, suffering from epilepsy for eight years. Cured in three months by S., third dilution.

6.—A poor lady's-maid, living at Pau; after uterine cauterization to relieve the pain of too difficult labour, the monthly period stopped, and, as a result, she was seized with convulsions, occurring eight or ten times a day. This lasted for seven years, and she became imbecile in consequence. There was evidently a diseased blood change. She had A., first dilution. The first day there was no attack; during the following week the attacks were less violent; the ninth day a bad attack. Then the dose was diminished, and she had the third dilution. Gradually the patient was cured. When forty-seven years old her periods returned, after being absent for more than seven years. And then she was cured.

7.—A man of 35, during the last two years, has had epileptic attacks, returning two or three times every month. Constitution much enfeebled by syphilis. Cure by Ven. alternately with A.; at first, third dilution; subsequently, ordinary doses.

Spinal Disease. 1.—Madame T. P., aged 50, confined to her bed for five years, and was unable to perform the most simple movements, in consequence of spinal inflammation. In addition to this, she had painful joints and varicose ulcerations on the legs. After having in vain tried all the known resources of allopathy and homœopathy, she was given up by all the professional attendants. She was completely cured by the following treatment:—Dilution S. alt. E., alt. A.; unctions of C^5 to the dorsal spine; then W. E. and B. E., with baths of C^5 alt. with A^2.

2.—Mr T. R., aged 62, had suffered for three years with terrible spinal disease and creeping paralysis. He had been given up as incurable by the most distinguished physicians, for his condition had become almost hopeless. Nevertheless, he wished to try the Mattei remedies. He was entirely cured by A. alt. S., first dilution; unctions of S^5 to the dorsal spine; W. E. and B. to the related nerves; baths of S., alternately with A^2. After two months' treatment he could walk; after five months he was entirely cured.

3.—Mr. N. M., aged 45, has had spinal disease for three years. All allopathic measures had been ineffectual. After treatment for one year with S. alt. A., and baths of the same remedies, he was perfectly cured.

4.—A young man of 21, could not hold himself upright on account of dislocation of a dorsal vertebra. Cured by S. in dilution, and external application of W. E.; also compresses of S.

5.—A child of 5 years had curvature of the dorsal spine, consequent upon fever. Cured by S., and external use of R. E. to each side of the dorsal spine.

ERYSIPELAS. 1.—From poison. December 15, 1881, a poor man, by trade a mechanic, accidentally introduced a splinter of brass into one of his fingers. Although the metal did not remain any length of time in the flesh, the whole arm became in a short time swollen; then the head; and this swelling was attended with horrible pains, intense fever, and delirium. The doctor who was called in, looking upon the case as desperate, gave no hope. S., first dilution, with R. E. to the nerve points of the arm and head, with unctions of S., promptly took down the swelling. In a few hours serious symptoms were confined to the injured part, which remained swollen and painful. For a week this treatment was continued, night and day, after which the arm was covered by a vesicular eruption, discharging a great quantity of serous fluid. It was a singular thing that whenever the use of R. E. was neglected, the swelling, as well as the delirium, returned actively, but subsided as soon as the R. E. was used.

This was the second accident of the same kind happening to the same man.

The first time the symptoms were less severe, and yet allopathic treatment had to be continued for three months before the case was disposed of; and then the surgeon was required to open a lymphatic gland in the armpit, which was considerably swollen. It was doubtless owing to this operation that several tendons were cut, and the unfortunate patient lost the use of his limb permanently. It was to be expected that he would select a different treatment when the same disease returned the other side.

2.—Mr. N. G., aged 58, was suffering from diffused erysipelas with general desquamation of the skin. He was cured by the internal use of S.

3.—Mr. V. M. of Dalmatia, aged 60, was attacked by grave heart distress and erysipelas. He was cured in three months by the internal use of A.

4.—Miss M. P., aged 17, had erysipelas. Was cured in a few days by S. internally, and the application of W. E. to the centre of the scalp.

Elephantiasis. 1.—C. F., aged 19, suffering from severe elephantiasis of the right leg. Treated internally by S. alt. A.; externally by baths of C^5 and all the electricities. She was cured in thirteen months.

2.—C. F., with elephantiasis on the right side. Cured by the C. and A. remedies internally and externally, in the course of three months.

3.—B. A., aged 50; elephantiasis of the right leg for two years. Cured by S. alt. E., alt. A., internally and externally.

4.—A young man, aged 16, had all the appearance of decrépit old age; his skin entirely covered with scales, like the skin oι an elephant, with numerous openings. C. and S. almost cured him; there remained only one opening with scales on the leg, but being impatient of treatment he took enormous doses, more and more strong, till he had taken two thousand globules daily. He was attacked by chest disease and died.

5.—A woman, aged 45, with elephantiasis in the right leg. Cured in fifteen months by unctions of L. alt. S., and compresses of S^5.

6.—A man, aged 50, with elephantiasis of the left leg. Was cured by S. alt. C.; compresses of G. E. and of S^5.

Hœmoptysis: or, spitting of blood; a case of relapse after two years. Cured in six months by A. internally. After five years there was no return.

Eczema.—Mr. P. N., suffering from eczema of the arms and buttocks. Cured L. alt. S^5.

Stomach Disease.—C. F., aged 52, was suffering from slow

gastritis, and declared incurable by several doctors. Nevertheless, S. internally, and unctions of F^2, were effectual in restoring him to health.

CARDIALGIA. 1.—Neuralgia of the stomach. A woman, aged 32, suffering from cardialgia with epigastric suffering, and pain in the back and chest. S. alt. A., second dilution: application of R. E. alt. Y. E., and some drops of Y. E. introduced by hypodermic injection, allayed the epigastric pain. The pains in the back and chest, however, only yielded to unctions of F^2 and application of W. E. After a week jaundice appeared, and this, with all the other symptoms, finally ceased under the action of F., second dilution, and unctions of F^2 to the hypochondria.

2.—P. R., aged 27, suffering for a fortnight from cardialgia and gastric catarrh. After some days he was cured by S^5 and F., second dilution, and external use of R. E. But, a month later, a very serious relapse occurred, which would not yield to these remedies. The ash-coloured evacuations showed liver complications. He was then treated by F. alt. A., second dilution, and unctions of F^2 to the hypochondria; and at the end of a week the cure was complete.

FEVERS. 1.—A brother of the Ecoles Chrétiennes, in Africa, aged 54, was taken with intermittent fever in 1868, and it remained regularly in paroxysms up to July, 1881. During the last five months, the attacks, which had become quotidian, assumed a pernicious character in spite of the bitters and quinine which he had taken in doses amounting to more than twenty grains a day.

The increase of the disease and the over use of medicines had produced the following condition: Acute gastric pains for two years, colic, disordered sight (diplopia, triplopia), kidney disease, dysuria, almost complete paralysis of the right arm for four months, sores with abundant oozing, excessive itching of the armpits, the hamstring hollows, and the bend of the elbow, very painful contractions in the diaphragm. The excessive irritation over all parts of the body having caused such emaciation in a few weeks as to reduce the patient almost to a skeleton, was produced by parasitic insects all over the body.

Of two medical gentleman who were called in, one declared that he could not make out the character of the disease; the other that it was unimportant, simply neuralgia. However, the patient at last could neither lie down nor compose himself to sleep, nor even lean back in his arm-chair without convulsive fainting attacks.

Treatment began July 1. Ver., first dilution, 10 globules dry and compresses of the same, 20 globules to a glass, under the armpits, behind the knees, in the forearms, and over the abdomen. F., second dilution. Compresses and unctions of F^2 on the hypochondria, the kidneys, and on the paralyzed arm. R. E. alt. Y. E. on the arm, the kidneys, the sub- and supra-orbital regions, three times a day; the same on the stomach. 2 globules of F. and 2 of C^5, dry, daily.

On the 15th, nephritis was sensibly diminished; normal vision had returned, the oozing and itching disappeared. Diarrhœa of inky colour; and formation of a phlegmonous abscess on the right side of the stomach; this was owing to the decomposition of retained worms.

On the 22nd, the opening of the abscess, there was an enormous discharge of sero-purulent matter mixed with altered blood, nearly three pints. The condition of the patient was very grave. He could take no nourishment; abundant perspirations; there was a cadaverous odour pervading the room and even beyond, and the characteristic signs of an impending fatal issue in the features. The doctor, called for the third time, declared that the patient had lost all his vitality and had not more than forty-eight hours of life in him.

The same treatment was continued, except Ver.; the dilutions were the third. R. E. alt. Y. E. five times a day. A lotion of brandy with C^6, 20 globules to the glass, on the vertebral column. Compresses of the same on the forehead and temples.

The cure was effected in two months. Fever has not returned; the appetite is good, the digestion excellent, and his strength is not unlike that which belonged to him ten years before.

2. Tertian Fever.—Madame E. de W., aged 30, was about to return to Russia, her native country, when she was taken with tertian ague, which is so terrible a disease in Rome. After the second paroxysm she sent for me, asking me to cure her without quinine. On May 17, 1881, she took F., second dilution; but I could not induce her to apply F^2 to the hypochondria. Nevertheless, by the 22nd of May, she was cured, that is in six days.

Cases of cure of intermittent fevers, both recent and of long standing and obstinate character, are innumerable. (*Dr. Held.*)

3. PUERPERAL FEVER. — Madame G. V., aged 20, suffering from puerperal and miliary fever. Cured by F. alt. A., alt. S., internally, and unctions of F^2 to the hypochondria.

4. INTERMITTENT FEVER.—E. Z., aged 28, had suffered for several months from ague. In five days he was cured by F. in dilution, and unctions of F^2 to the hypochondria.

5. SCARLET FEVER.—A woman, aged 26, attacked by scarlatina, with rash all over the body, was cured in four days by S^2, in dilution, and unctions of F^2 to the hypochondria.

Dr. Atzninger, during the month of May, 1882, when scarlatina prevailed at Vienna, had many prompt and brilliant cures by the use of F. and S. alternately, and unctions of F^2 to the hypochondria.

6. SMALL-POX.—A little girl, aged 3, was attacked with variola; the Mattei remedies were not employed till the eruption was complete. Treatment, S. alt. F., second dilution ; 1 globule of S. dry every half-hour, and a teaspoonful of the dilution every ten minutes. Tepid compresses of S^5 on the pustules. The fever was immediately arrested. The next day the eruption was dried up as if some therapeutic frost had nipped them in the bud.

7. FEVER.—Mr. J. D., in consequence of fevers which remained hanging over him for five years, was troubled with serious disorder in the viscera of the hypochondrium, especially the liver. For five years he resorted to all kinds of allopathic remedies, without result. Then he was cured in a single month by taking F. in dilution, and the application of F^2 unctions to the hypochondria.

8. FEVER.—Rev. P. J., Procurator-general of the Capucin order, reports that he had suffered from fever for a considerable time. After the use of F. in dilution and in unctions, the fever disappeared.

FISTULA : *Lachrymalis fistula.*—1. Mr. S., aged 30, had lachrymal fistula in the right eye. He was given local washes and lotions of S. alternately with W. E. and S. internally. The cure was complete.

2. LACHRYMAL FISTULA in the left eye, in a man aged 22. Cured by S. alternately with A. Local applications of S^5 alternately with C^5, and W. E.

3. Dental Fistula.—E. C., aged 10, cheek so much swollen that he could not open his mouth, caused by dental fistula, and the gum infiltrated with matter. His pains were unendurable. He was ordered L., second dilution; compresses and gargles of the same. The next day the swelling was reduced; the fistula had discharged an immense quantity of matter, and after two days' treatment the child was cured by L. alone.

4. Anal Fistula.—Madame A., aged 32, suffered from fistula ani, and uterine inflammation. She was completely cured in three months by the alternation of C. and A., first dilution; 6 globules of S. dry, daily; and alternate baths of C^5 and A^2, 100 globules to the bath. She also had compresses of R. E and G. E. to the affected parts. The lady was not only cured, but declared that she had never been so well in health.

5. Anal Fistula.—V. L., aged 39, had fistula ani, with much pain and suppuration. Being unwilling to submit to a surgical operation, and having exhausted, without result, all the resources of allopathy, he resolved to try the Mattei remedies, as an almost hopeless expedient. Nevertheless, he was cured in four months by alternation of S. and L. at ordinary doses, application of R. E. to the sacrum, baths and compresses of C^5 locally.

Liver cases. 1.—L. R., aged 18, suffering from hepatitis—inflammation of the liver—was entirely cured in three weeks by F. alternately with A^3, third dilution. Compresses to the hypochondria, kept up night and day, with F^2 and W. E.

2.—G. P., aged 48, suffering for some years with severe disorder of the liver. He had been obliged almost every year to resort to Vichy for the waters. These always brought some relief, but the evil always returned, and even with augmented severity, never leaving him entirely free. For the last three months the patient was suffering from intermittent fever, of unusual severity, over which quinine seemed to have no influence.

He began Electro-Homœopathic treatment January 1, 1880, after a violent paroxysm of fever; he took F. in the second dilution, and unctions of F^2 over the hypochondria. The fever only returned once, and on the 15th of Febuary the patient appeared restored to his normal state. However, it was deemed prudent to continue the use of remedies for some time, and the liver disease entirely disappeared.

3.—Madame N. L., aged 40, suffering from most agonizing hepatic colic. By the use of F., and compresses of F^2, these sufferings rapidly ceased.

4.—Chronic congestion of the liver and spleen, consequent upon repeated attacks of tertian ague, and abuse of quinine. Mr. A. P., aged 58, has been liable every spring, since he was 15 years old, to attacks of tertian ague, which have always been suppressed by large doses of quinine. The result is a considerable enlargement of the liver and spleen. Under pressure the liver feels hard; he has a jaundiced tint, the root of the tongue is coated yellow, taste bitter and clammy, bowels disturbed. His mood is changeable, melancholic, irritated by the least contradiction, he sees everything in gloomy lights. In short, his temper is typically hypochondriacal.

In 1881, January 6, he took F. in the second dilution, and used F^2 externally to the hypochondria night and morning: also 1 globule, dry, of S. night and morning, gradually the doses of F. were increased up to the strength of the first dilution.

After a month's treatment on this plan, the patient's complexion changed; jaundice ceased, and the yellow coating on the tongue became white. His mood also was considerably improved, and his digestion became easier; but there was no palpable alteration in the condition of the liver and spleen. Nevertheless, I did not change the treatment, for in such a short ime there could not be any very notable improvement in the congested viscera.

In the month of March, Mr. A. P., began to feel the usual premonitory symptoms of his habitual spring ague. Rather disappointed, he asked me whether he ought not to take a few decisive doses of quinine, in order to suppress the threatening fever. I answered decidedly, No! and made him take F. in the third instead of the first dilution, while continuing persistently unctions of F^2 to the hypochondria, and R. E. to the sympathetic nerve and solar plexus. At the end of two days all the symptoms of approaching fever, except a *malaise*, had left him. F. in the second dilution disposed of all the remaining symptoms, and on the fourth day, Mr. A. P. returned to the first dilution in F., without having required the assistance of quinine, which had been indispensible under allopathic regime.

In the month of August, I ascertained that the liver as well as the spleen was entirely free from the congestion which had lasted so many years. But, although cured, I begged Mr. A. P. to continue the use of F., internally and externally, till the end of the year, in order to consolidate his cure. He did this, and remained well.

This case proves the great influence which F. exerts on disorders of the liver and spleen, and on all forms of intermittent fever: also its efficacy as an antidote to quinine, and to remove the ill effects of its long continued use. (*Dr. Held.*)

5. Chronic Hepatitis.—R. J., aged 50, having been till three years since under allopathic treatment, was cured in two months by F. in dilution, and unctions of F^2 to the hypochondria.

6.—Mr. P. P., aged 56, suffered from grave liver affection, with hæmorrhage. He was cured in three weeks by A. in dilution, and unctions of F^2 to the hypochondria.

Weakness of the Arms from a fall.—Absolute inability to lift the arm, and even to bring the hand to the chest. Removed by the external use of R. E.

Weakness of the Knees.—Cured by S. and S. used alternately, and application of R. E. to the crural and sciatic nerves—the application being made to the neighbourhood of the knee.

Facial Neuralgia.—Two cases, cured by S. in the first dilution, and the external application of R. E. alternately with Y. E.

Another case of facial neuralgia, of intermittent type, cured by S. alternately with F., application of R. E. and unctions of F^2 to the hypochondria.

Fracture of the Jaw.—A man, aged 34, cured by S. internally and externally, and compresses of W. E. After twenty days' treatment, he again returned to Count Mattei for inspection, and he ascertained that the two parts of the bone were solidly united.

Cases of Knee Disease.—1. White swelling. A. Bonditi, a woman of Savignan, aged 21, was suffering from white swelling of the knee, with caries of the bone, and two suppurating openings. She was treated for two years by the A. and C. remedies, in dilution, and alternate applications of R. E. and Y. E. She was completely cured.

2.—Lymphatic swelling of the knee. Madame R. M. had been suffering for fifteen years from a lymphatic swelling of the right knee. After six months' treatment by A. alternately with S. and C., internally and externally, she was entirely cured.

3.—Madame F., aged 40, had white swellings on the articulations of the lower limbs, dating from the age of five years. She was cured by C. alternately with A., and unctions of the same remedies.

4.—A young man had for several years been suffering from anchylosis of the knee, with a hard tumour underneath; and could not walk without a crutch. He was cured in two months by S., internally, with compresses and unctions of the same remedy externally.

5.—Swelling of the knee resulting from difficult labour. The infant was still-born, and had an enormous hydrocephalic head. The mother, aged 47, was remarkably angioitic. Treatment by A. alternately with C. was continued at all doses, without success, for two or three months. The following prescription was then adopted: Ven. F. C. A. S. in weak doses. Three months after, the tumour, which was as large as two united fists, hard, and apparently requiring surgical interference, was much reduced; and some weeks later it had completely disappeared, leaving no traces of its former existence or removal.

6.—Swelling of the knee and caries of the bone. Mr. F. B., a young man, aged 23, had suffered from rheumatism in the left leg since the age of four years. A swelling had appeared on the right knee, as well as an enormous ganglion under the articulation; moreover, the limb was generally much atrophied. Six months before, severe pain set in, followed by dull and continued pain, indicative of caries of the bone. At the hospital the surgeons told him that it would be necessary to remove two portions of the bone; but before anæsthesia was produced, they wished him to authorize them to amputate the limb if they should consider it necessary. Inferring from this that they did so consider, he refused treatment, and in despair sent to me, begging me to treat him with the Mattei remedies, this being his last resource. I prescribed C. in the second dilution, unctions of C^5, W. E. applied night and morning, constant compresses during the day of C^5, application of R. E. alt. Y. E. along the crural nerve. Marked improvement set in in a few days. Three weeks afterwards, I gave C^5 internally, and 2 globules dry of S. night and morning. Since that time the man blesses untiringly the venerated name of Count Mattei. He can walk eight or nine miles daily without fatigue and without pain. The tumour has disappeared, the ganglion and atrophie are arrested. For a considerable time he continued the treatment in order to avoid any relapse of such a serious disease, and especially in order to destroy the last germs of the disease. (*S. Schmidt.*)

Cases of Gangrene. 1.—S. S., aged 79, living at Bologna, was afflicted with cutaneous gangrene on the right eyelid. This had been treated with caustics, and was cured in a short time by baths of C.

2.—G. R., aged 17, had frontal gangrene over the right orbit, caused by contusions. The gangrenous ulceration was caused by the internal use of C.

3.—F. G., aged 66. Injury to the face, consequent upon a fall, with ulceration and threatened gangrene. He was perfectly cured in a fortnight by C^5 in dilution, alternately with A. Compresses, alternating, of the same remedies, and the use of B. E.

4.—Mr. G. F., aged 50, had a gangrenous ulcer on the nostrils, pronounced incurable. He was cured in two months by S. alt. A., alt. C., internally and externally.

5.—Gangrene of the foot. Wounded joint. Amputation determined upon. The foot was already black. Cured in six months by C. internally and externally.

6.—Gangrene of the arm, after amputation some time before, in a man aged 23. Cured by C. internally and externally.

Gout.—Mr. L. P., aged 55, Major domo at Briganzia, had suffered from gout for five years; was cured by S., internally and externally, and compresses of G. E. to the joints.

Throat Inflammation.—Mrs. R. P., aged 27, suffering from angina; was completely cured by C. internally, and compresses of W. E.

Disease of the Glands. 1.—A little girl, aged 3, with her head covered with scab and indurations, was treated with S. internally. An enormous glandular swelling appeared on the neck, near the ear. The treatment was S. and C. internally, unctions of C, and application of G. E. The child is now well, lively, perfectly cured.

2.—Miss E. R,, aged 12, suffered from general glandular disease of a serious character. She was cured by C. internally, and unctions of the same remedy.

3.—Mr. G. J., aged 30, had suffered from inflamed parotid glands for some months. Was perfectly cured by C. internally, and unctions of C^5.

4.—Ulcerated cervical glands. A little girl, aged 6, very scrofulous, with suppurating ears, large ulcer on the back, unconquerable repugnance to meat, and even for all kinds of food. In a few weeks all the wounds had cicatrized, the appetite and strength returned, and the whole condition improved greatly. The medicine was S.

Goitre. 1.—A young girl, aged 15, had a very prominent thyroid gland, which distressed her extremely. Cure was effected in two months, and all deformity removed by S. alternately with A. and S., first dilution. Unctions of C^5 and R. E. by cupping.

2.—A man, aged 26, cured by F. alternately with C. in the first dilution. Unctions of C^5 and application of R. E. in compresses around the gland.

Ganglion.—A lady, aged 60, for six or eight months had had a growth on the wrist as large as a hazel nut. The doctor whom she consulted told her that it was a ganglion, and that the sole means of dispersing it was by crushing—which might be a little painful. The lady decided to try electro-homeopathy. She applied compresses of C^5 to the affected wrist, constantly renewed, night and day; using 15 globules to a glass of water. In less than three days the ganglion entirely disappeared, and has not returned.

Hæmorrhoids.—Mr. H. Pontontoff, 40, of St. Petersburg, had suffered for fifty years from bleeding hæmorrhoids, with enlargement of the liver; palpitation of the heart, its action being at the rate of about 120 beats a minute; loss of appetite, and great weakness. All allopathic remedies had proved unsuccessful. After ten days' treatment with A^3 alt. F^1, alt. C^1, second dilution, and 10 globules of S. dry daily. Unctions on the heart of A^2, and F^2 on the hypochondria alt. C^5, produced immense and increasing relief, and after two months a complete cure was the result.

Hysteria.—Mrs. A. L., aged 26, had suffered from hysterical convulsions for six years. She was cured in ten days by C. in dilution, and unctions of the same remedy on the stomach.

1. Herpes.—Mrs. F. A., with herpes in the arm, chest, and the lower part of the stomach, with arthritic pains; was cured in two months by S. internally, and in compresses.

2. Herpes.—Professor de Micheles, aged 46, having suffered for 16 years from herpes, was cured by A. internally, after four months' treatment.

1. Hernia.—Mrs. B. S., aged 42, had suffered for a year from a very large hernia in the left groin. After five months' treatment with A. in dilution, and local baths of R. E., she was cured.

Hysteria.—Mrs. R. V., aged 49, suffered for seven years from chronic hysteria. After four months' treatment with S. internally she was cured.

2. Hernia.—Mr. F. S., aged 27, suffered from left inguinal hernia. He was cured by the internal use of S^1, without any other medicine.

1. Dropsy (Ovarian Ascites).—Mrs. P. R., aged 55, had been confined to her bed for a long time with ovarian disease and dropsy, and was given up as incurable. Yielding to the urgent request of the poor woman, I left her several doses of S. and C., to be alternated in the second dilution, with compresses and unctions of C^5 and S^5; this was the 25th of March. On the 14th of April the stomach was, to her great astonishment, much less swollen, and was like that of a woman after confinement. The water of the ovarian cyst had been discharged with the urine. I encouraged her to continue perseveringly a treatment which had begun so favourably. On the 18th of June, as the progress of improvement was somewhat arrested, I gave C. alt. with Ven., and compresses of C^1 alt. S^5, after which the progress of recovery was uninterrupted; it continued in a more and more marked degree until August, when the patient was considered radically cured. Four years have passed without showing any return of this terrible disease. *Note.*—With reference to the use of Ven. in disorders of the ovaries and uterus, I may observe that, as a rule, all these maladies, including leucorrhœa (which, perhaps, in these cases is only chronic gonorrhœa), when they resist C. carried up to the third dilution, yield to Ven., either alone or in alternation with C. From this I conclude that constitutional syphilis in women; always starting in the uterus, which is the seat of many diseases, is not so rare a disease as one might imagine. In every ten cases of uterine disease, manifested either by megrim, or by leucorrhœa, four are most easily cured by Ven. Whatever may be the explanation, my opinion

is that Ven. has the properties of either S. or C., which might explain these cases; at any rate, I have always had recourse to this kind of treatment for the diseases in question. Not only when they resist, but when also the action of C. is simply too slow, I alternate Ven., and with good results.

2. Dropsy (Ascites).—A young girl. Considerable swelling of the abdomen, produced by enlargement of the mesenteric glands, with great emaciation. Cured radically by C.

3. Tuguinal Hernia.—A man, aged 60, of feeble constitution, suffering for fifteen years from hernia, with varices, and incompetency of the valves of the heart. Cured with S. alt. A.

4. Tuguinal Hernia.—A girl, aged 11, suffering from headache, indigestion, &c.; a hernia of the size of a pigeon's egg was discovered. S., first dilution, was given, and R. E. around the hernia. After forty-five days the position of the hernia could no longer be recognized by touch. The use of S. was continued for six months by way of precaution, and cure was complete. She was cured in three months, with complete cicatrization of the ulcers, by second dilutions of A., C., and S., used alternately. Powdered globules of S. alternately with W. E. were applied to the larynx. Application of B. E. to the sympathetic, the solar plexus, the occiput, and the pit of the stomach.

2. Laryngeal Catarrh.—Mr. P. had suffered for a long time from laryngeal catarrh. He was completely cured by first dilutions of S. and A. alternately, with unctions and gargles of the same remedies to the throat and neck.

3. Laryngitis with Croupy Cough.—A little girl, aged 4, was suddenly taken, about midnight, with a frightful cough, resembling a cock-crowing, and with all the premonitory symptoms of false croup. She was immediately given one globule of P., one of S., and one of Ven. At the same time cupping applications of R. E. were made on the great hypoglossi, and she was made to gargle with the same electricity, ten drops to a glass of water. After an hour the state of the child was no longer grave. She had, however, for four or five hours every ten minutes, a teaspoonful of P. in dilution, or a globule of P^3 or of S. The next day the child was so far recovered that it could rise. She continued to take S. and P. alternately in dilution for two days, as a safeguard against relapse.

Dislocation of the Foot.—A young girl, aged 18, dislocated

her foot some years before. At first not much notice was taken of it; accordingly it became worse, and a wound was formed on the ankle so that she could not put her foot to the ground. The doctor in attendance wished her to be removed to the hospital, and submit to amputation. The mother, however, wished to try the Mattei remedies; and the girl was cured by dilutions of S. and C^3 taken alternately, and compresses alternately of S^2 and B. E.

LUPUS. 1.—G. M., aged 22, had lupus, extending over the face. By the use of C., the disease was reduced to a case of simple nasal ulceration. Treatment was continued.

LUPUS. 2.—Another case was a woman, aged 21, who had suffered from the same disease for four years. She was completely cured by C., S., and A., used both internally and externally.

LUPUS. 3.—Marie Mazzotti, aged 37; had never observed any venereal disease. Suddenly she was attacked by a large sore on the face, which involved the eyes, the nose, and the forehead, and, having caused loss of the hair, filled the scalp with scurf. Mr. Gamerini, of Bologna, treated the case allopathically for three years without result. Neither iodine nor mercury improved the condition of the patient in any degree, and, after these three years, she was given up as incurable. A year afterwards, that is the fourth year of the disease, she was treated by Ven. internally and externally; and, after six months, this suffering woman regained her natural features; the eyes and nose were saved, the sore disappeared, the hair began to grow again. She was cured.

LEUCORRHŒA. 1.—Mrs. R. A., aged 34, had suffered for a year with leucorrhœa, attended with terrible pain in the abdomen. She was cured in a short time by the first dilutions alternately of L. and A.; compresses of A^2 over the heart; abdominal compresses and injections of L.

LEUCORRHŒA. 2.—A lady, aged 37, married, had leucorrhœa, with uterine pain and daily attacks. She was cured in a few days by C. internally, and unctions of C^5 over the abdomen.

5. HERNIA.—A man, aged 69, had suffered from hernia for seven years. At times he suffered severely; he was always constipated, and wore a support, which annoyed him excessively. At first A. in the first dilution was given, and the constipation

ceased in three days; after that treatment was continued with C., alternately with A^3. Compresses of B. E. over the hernia. The support was entirely discontinued, and in a month a radical cure was effected.

6. HERNIA.—R. D., aged 14, threatened with right inguinal hernia, had a wound in the locality caused by the friction of the truss. Moreover, he was troubled with weakness of sight and burning in the eyes. The wound was cured by C^5 and B. E. The sight was improved by baths of A^2 and applications of W. E.

7. UMBILICAL HERNIA.—A lady, aged 52, suffering for two years, was cured in five months by S., in first dilution, and compresses of R. E.

8. DROPSY, OVARIAN.—Madame G. J., aged 35, had chronic ovarian inflammation, and, moreover, was pregnant for six months. After taking C. internally, and using unctions of C^5 externally, the disease was vanquished, and a favourable confinement followed.

4. DROPSY.—Madame P., aged 25, suffered from dropsy, caused by obstruction of the liver and spleen, pronounced incurable. She was perfectly cured by A. internally, and unctions of F^2 to the hypochondria.

INDIGESTION.—A lady, suffering from chronic humming in the ears, with headache and chronic indigestion, was cured in two months by A^2, second dilution. Unctions of A^2 over the heart and around the ears, and of L. over the head.

INTESTINAL INFLAMMATION.—A woman, aged 36, suffered from intestinal inflammation so acutely that pelvic movement was almost impossible. She was cured by S., alternately with C^5, first dilution, and unctions of C^5 to the abdomen and loins.

INTOXICATION AND LEAD POISONING, in a man of 60, arose by the dissolving in wine of lead shot which had been used to clean the bottles, and which had not been carefully removed before refilling and sealing the bottles. The poisoning took place at Tamatava, in Madagascar, in June and July, 1882.

The first attack occurred on the 15th of July. As the poisoning had been slow, the patient lost his reason, and became furious. The doctor of the town was able to calm down the furious symptoms, but could not restore either the reason or the strength, which had disappeared with the attack. Nor could he succeed in saving the patient's fellow-sufferer from the same cause, aged 56, who died after sixty hours of intense suffering. On the 20th of July the patient arrived at the Reunion Isle, and on the 3rd of August there was a fresh attack, for which the best doctors in the island could do nothing effectual. The patient, when out walking, was suddenly seized with convulsions, and became stiffened and fixed to the spot. Two hours afterwards, violent spasms in all the limbs, loss of speech, very severe oppression of the breath, mucous rales, complete immobility, abdominal distension, generally cataleptic and inflexible state. The next day I was sent for at eight in the evening. Treatment began as follows: ten globules of S^5, dry, every half-hour, and a small teaspoonful of the second dilution of S^5, alternately with A^2, every five minutes, the mouth being kept slightly open by means of a strong iron plate. Every five minutes cupping applications of R. E., alternately with Y. E., to the solar plexus, occiput, and great sympathetic. On account of violent perspiration, frequent compresses of F^2, alternately with S^5 and A^2, fifteen globules to a glassful of water.

Unctions every half-hour on the temples, the root of the nose, the cranial sutures, and on the vertex of the head, of S^5, alternately with A^3, four globules to a tablespoonful, with the addition of a few drops of W. E. Next day, at two in the morning, respiration was more free, the rales intermittent and weaker. The treatment is reduced to the use of the unctions at hourly intervals. After six in the morning, compresses on the head and abdomen are continued, and sipping occasionally. The rales became more continuous and stronger than on the preceding day. There was an offensive odour, reaching even to the antechamber. On Saturday night and on Sunday same compresses only were applied. I no longer dared hope for any success. On Sunday, at five or six in the morning, the limbs again became flexible, the rales were not continuous; a gangrenous odour exhaled from the mouth. The former treatment was resumed. Nevertheless, the sipping could not be continued, for the six or eight drops of water which were placed on the tongue passed into the windpipe, and provoked a long drum-like rumbling. From eight to ten o'clock the eyes were half open, dull, faded, turned upwards, insensible to light or heat; then the cornea became red and livid; the orbits swollen, first livid, then almost black. At ten the patient uttered piteous cries, and at the same time struck himself repeatedly over the ribs; there was a sudden outbreak of large patches, the size of a penny, over the surface of the chest and around the heart, perspiration of bloody tint from the pit of the stomach to the forehead, so free that it could be wiped off with a cloth. With a view of re-establishing respiration, at six o'clock in the morning, I applied over the sympathetic, near the collar-bone, compresses made of six globules of S^5, and five drops of R. E. to a tablespoonful of water. From noon till eight in the evening the paroxysms of cries and striking on the chest were redoubled, as before. The last paroxysm was like a child calling out, "Mamma! mamma!" Urination also occurred twice. Speech did not yet return. The next day, W. E. and compresses of S^5; B. E. over the hypoglossi. At the end of two days speech became almost normal; a week afterwards the expression of the face was calm and pleasing. An enema daily of S^5, alternately with A^2, fifteen globules; washes three times a day of brandy and C. over the vertebral column to bring back strength; this was effected in three weeks. S^5, alternately with A^3, fifteen globules in the glass of water, was used externally on the temples, the forehead, the occiput, and the head three times a day, in order to restore mental power. In five weeks the patient was completely cured. Moreover, he is rid of *delirium tremens*, to which he had been liable for the last two years, in consequence of a too free use of alcohol.

Cysts. 1.—Madame M., aged 40, suffering for two years from right-sided ovarian cysts, irregular palpitation, and congestion of the liver. Was cured in ten months by the second dilutions, taken in alternation, of A., F., and C.; unctions of F^2 to the hypochondria; unctions of C^5 over the region where the cyst is detected, and applications of W. E. to the sympathetic, the occiput, the solar plexus, and the pit of the stomach.

Cysts. 2.—Madame L. R., aged 48, with ovarian cysts; abdomen full of fluid, emaciation, constant cough, febrile state. The allopathic attendants at Vienna affirmed that there was no remedy but operation. She had Mattei treatment as follows: Second dilution of C., unctions and compresses of C^5 over the abdomen, applications of R. E. to the great sympathetic, the solar plexus, the occiput, and pit of the stomach. After eight weeks the cyst was much smaller, and six months afterwards the lady was completely cured.

Chronic Laryngitis.—Miss P., aged 22, suffering from chronic laryngeal ulceration, voice damaged, burning pains, painful deglutition, purulent expectoration, evening fever, cough, offensive breath. Cauterization had been repeatedly employed; the disease was not touched by allopathic treatment.

Leucorrhœa. 3.—Miss A., aged 23, had suffered from leucorrhœa for four years, with loss of appetite, dyspepsia, and pains in the lower limbs. She was cured in six months by the second dilutions, taken alternately, of C. and S.; W. E. to the perinæum, pubes, and sacrum. Unctions of C^5, applications of Y. E., and baths of C^5.

Uterine Cases.

Metrorrhagia. 1.—Miss H. suffered for a year from metrorrhagia. She had exhausted all ordinary medical resources; among other things a three months' course of arsenic. By Electro-Homœopathy she was cured in five days. The following was the treatment: First dilutions of A^3 and C. alternately; unctions of F^2 to the hypochondria, of A^3 over the heart, and of C^5 over the abdomen. Five globules of S., dry, at mealtimes.

2.—Madame J., aged 44, with metrorrhagia of seven months' standing; was cured in three months by A. in dilution, and three drops of B. E. on sugar daily.

3.—A girl, aged 14, had metrorrhagia, with violent pains; was promptly cured by the second dilution of A., and compresses of A. over the abdomen.

Prolapsus Uteri, of two years' standing, with great emaciation, insomnia, violent pains in the kidney regions and the thighs, dysuria, frequent vomiting of greenish matters; was cured in two months by C. in dilution, unctions of C., and application of R. E. to the great sympathetic, the solar plexus, and the pit of the stomach.

2.—Prolapsus uteri, which had resisted treatment by C., in the second dilution, with one globule of S., dry, night and morning, was cured by the first dilution of C. and A. alternately; eight globules of S., dry, *i.e.*, one every hour. Baths medicated by one hundred globules of C^5. Unctions of C^5 to the sacrum and the lower abdomen. Injections of A^2, twenty globules to the glass of water.

Polypus at the Os Uteri—In a woman, aged 67, three years

ago pronounced incurable. The tumour was in a few days reduced by C. internally, and the application of R. E. to the sacrum.

FIBROUS TUMOURS OF THE UTERUS, at the critical age. These were indicated by violent metrorrhagia, frequently returning, endangering life. The doctor used the usual allopathic expedients without much result. He then pronounced the case incurable, and gave the patient only a few weeks' life. A consultation of three of his colleagues confirmed this prognosis. The third dilutions of C. and A., with injections of C^5 and A^2, and applications of B. E., rapidly diminished the frequency and violence of the hæmorrhage. After four weeks a large quantity of quasi-vegitations were discharged. These tumours were carefully preserved by the doctor, till at last, finding that they continued to appear, he was obliged to think they were continually reproduced. The number of these vegetations was astonishing, and five doctors professed themselves perplexed by them. At the present time hæmorrhage returns only once a month, with slight hysteric paroxysms, and do not much differ from usual conditions. But if, as there is good reason to believe, improvement is maintained, cure will certainly arrive at last.

Another case.—A woman of 32, suffering from excessive hæmorrhages, was in danger of death from depletion. The doctor accounted for this by a fibrous tumour, on which he had operated several times, but which constantly returned after a short time. Hypodermic injections of ergotin, as well as of perchloride of iron, and painful and dangerous surgical operations, had been tried without result. Anemia was extreme, with venous murmur in the head. The patient could not leave her bed. In less than a fortnight external and internal treatment by A. and C. alternately (A^2 and C^5 externally) worked a veritable miracle. Hæmorrhage ceased. At the present time the patient is completely restored, to the great perplexity of the doctor.

MENINGITIS.—Baron A. B., of Vienna, aged 22, after feeling somewhat unwell for several days, became suddenly dangerously ill. He had terrible pains in the head, extending over the forehead and vertex; high fever; and elevated temperature. Under these circumstances my assistance was sought.

I found the patient delirious. I gave F. and S. alternately, internally. These, and compresses of W. E on the head, soon relieved the sufferings, broke the violence of the attack, and, in four days, established convalescence. After ten days the cure was complete.

Severe Injuries and Lacerations on the Head.—A nursing infant met with a severe fall from a window. The height was nearly twelve feet, and he sustained such severe injury to the head and right ribs that his condition was considered desperate and incurable. The appearance of strabismus (squinting) and coma, indicating approaching death, had also set in. After this prognosis was pronounced, the unhappy father, having scarcely a hope of saving his son, was fortunate enough to resort to Electro-Homœopathy, and his urgent desires were fulfilled, for after three weeks' treatment, with application of W. E., alternately with Y. E. and B. E., over the whole head, combined with the internal use of one globule, dry, of S., A^2, and C.—giving also at the same time and in the same order, second dilutions of the same to the mother—immediate improvement showed itself, and continued with increasing rapidity from day to day, so that, after three weeks, the infant was cured. It regained its mental faculties, which were almost entirely gone; and the sight, which was almost destroyed, returned. In a word, the cure was complete.

Mutism.—A woman of 45 was gradually affected by complete mutism. At first she had difficulty in articulation; then she could not produce more than isolated words; at length she could only say *yes* or *no*. For eighteen months she could not pronounce any word distinctly. Besides this, she had rheumatism in the arms. She had R. E. applied to the hypoglossi and to the nape of the neck for thirty seconds. During the minute afterwards she could say *yes* or *no*. By the use of S. she recovered speech in about a month.

Mutism.—Loss of speech, from fright, in a girl of 7, was cured by the application of R. E. to the occiput and the small hypoglossi.

Ozœna. 1.—A son of Mr. M., aged 11, was condemned to almost complete isolation in consequence of the offensive odour proceeding from the nose, and caused by chronic mucous ulceration, with loss of smell. He was cured by first dilution, used alternately, of S., C^4, and A^2; unctions and aspiration by the nostrils of C^4; applications of R. E., alternately with Y. E., to the related nerve centres.

Ozœna. 2.—A young woman had had scrofulous ozœna from infancy. She was treated by S., but had to discontinue treatment from time to time, owing to the pains in the nose which came on. Soon fragments of the ethmoid bone showed themselves in the nasal secretion, diminishing gradually till cure was completed.

Ozœna. 3.—A lady, aged 30, with a very lymphatic constitution, had suffered for two years from ozœna. The discharge was purulent, with a most offensive odour. Sixty handkerchiefs a week were not enough. She was cured in six months by S., and the applications of R. E. to the root of the nose and the occiput.

Neuralgia of the supra-orbital nerves, returning daily at the same hour, and resisting all treatment, was cured by F., in dilution, and unctions of F^2 to the hypochondria.

Nymphomania.—Miss L. B., suffering for thirteen years from nymphomania and chronic gastritis. She was cured in a short time by S. internally, and baths of C^5.

Nervous Disease.—Mrs. F. had suffered for about thirty years from a distressing nervous disease, reappearing at fixed intervals. Repeated fainting attacks, with violence, so that it took several persons to keep her in bed; after the paroxysms, great depression. The methods used for relief, such as purgatives, vesicants, &c., did little or no good.

On the death of her son, terrible paroxysms appeared; afterwards great weakness and inflammation in the abdomen. Treatment was begun by C. in the second dilution, and the inflammation was arrested in twenty-four hours. Improvement continued, but severe pains in the head remained, which ultimately yielded to C^3 in the second dilution. She had also applications of W. E., and compresses of C^5 over the head. B. E. took away the sciatic and crural pains, and restored strength. This lady continued the use of the electricity once daily, and the internal use of the second dilution of C^3. She is in moderately good health, and a perfect cure may be looked for in due time.

Nervous Paroxysms.—A young girl, aged 16, was subject every night to an attack of a nervous character, neither hysteric nor epileptic, affecting only the left side of the body and the limbs of the same side. Probably on account of the unusual character of these attacks, the only danger attaching to them arose from the sudden interference with circulation, causing severe determination of blood to the head. In her general state there was no serious vascular alteration. S., given first in the third, then in the first, dilution, produced no effect. Then she had Ver., one globule, dry, every hour. After two days the young girl passed a large quantity of thread worms. Since that the paroxysms have not returned.

Ear Cases. Deafness. 1.—R. G., aged 63, was deaf, especially in the right ear. In forty days he was perfectly cured by S.

2. Deficiency of Hearing.—Mr. P., aged 42, was cured by the first dilutions, alternately, of S. and A.; B. E. applied to the skull, to the small muscles behind the ear; and occasionally some drops of W. E. in the ear passages.

3. Deafness.—F. R., aged 44, deaf since the age of 18, was cured in four months by A. internally, and applications alternately of R. E. and Y. E. to the small muscles behind the ear.

4. Deafness.—A woman had been deaf for five years. She was cured in three months by C., alternately with S. and A., in dilution, and W. E. behind the ear.

5. Deafness.—A young soldier, having taken cold in his tent, suffered for eight months from violent pains in the head, running from the ear, and complete deafness on one side. He was completely cured in a fortnight by S., internally. He had also applications of R. E., and injections of S., fifteen globules to the glass.

Loss of Smell.—Loss of smell, resulting from a surgical operation on the forehead; it was restored in a few minutes by the use of R. E.

Bone Cases. 1. Exostosis.—Tumour on the periosteum of the right arm of a man, aged 27, was cured by S^2; the application of R. E. to the related nerve centres; compresses of C^5, and baths of the same remedy.

2. Exostosis on the right leg, in an old man, was cured in two months by S. internally and externally.

3. Spinal Ventosa and Foot Disease.—The patient had numerous sores on his leg of a citron colour, mucous membrane of the mouth diseased, excessive emaciation. The surgeons wished to amputate the leg, but the patient was thought too

weak, and the operation was abandoned. In three years he was cured, and he has enjoyed good health for eight years. The treatment was by S., by which the carious bone was expelled and the wound cicatrized.

4. FRACTURE.—O. A., aged 80, had fracture of her right knee-cap. But this was not all. While the fracture was being treated, a lymphatic tumour developed, and the knee joint was almost entirely anchylosed. The doctors attempted to cure it, but failed. The patient was then advised to go to Bologna, and to put herself under Count Mattei, who cured her in four months by C., alternately with A., externally and internally.

CASES OF PARALYSIS. 1. FACIAL.—Mr. D., aged 30, was suffering from facial paralysis on the left side, and treated at the hospital without result. He then had B. E. internally, and R. E. externally, and was cured in eighteen days.

PARALYSIS. 2. GENERAL.—Mrs. A., of London; paralysis of six years' standing. Her condition was serious and complicated. She could not, without great difficulty, raise her hands to her head; the knees and feet were benumbed. Several of the fingers and toes were still the seat of severe rheumatic pains and of calcareous deposit. The whole surface of the body, especially the head and the thighs, was covered with a thick coating of eczematous incrustations. The monthly function was very irregular, and always extremely painful.

I treated the patient with R. E., which soon restored function to the paralysed limbs. The C^5, which she took for four months consecutively, re-established healthy and painless monthly functions. Strength returned gradually under the action of Ven. and of S., and the skin regained all its smoothness and suppleness. For more than eighteen months this lady has enjoyed good health. She now walks between two and three miles.

PARALYSIS. 3.—Of the left leg, from typhoid fever. L., aged 14, had been ill since the age of two. His leg was literally dried up; he had no muscles and no calf. The limb was so contracted that the great toe could scarcely touch the ground. No treatment had been of any avail, although the child had been treated by the most distinguished surgeons in London.

We employed daily baths of R. E. with S. internally. At the end of five months, this young man had made such astonishing progress that the leg had regained its natural state. The muscles were developed, the weakness of the dorsal spine had disappeared, and, ultimately, the young man could plant his foot firmly on the ground, and enjoyed excellent health.

PARALYSIS. 4.—Of the left side. Cured in three weeks. Mr. R. aged 58, of robust constitution, inclined to cerebral congestion, had had two slight apoplectic attacks over a period of two years, without very serious results. At the beginning of last year Mr. R. had another attack, this time a more violent one, leaving entire paralysis of the left side.

I saw the patient one hour after the attack. He was in bed, and unable to turn or to make the slightest movement of the arm or leg, or to bend the fingers of the left hand. The face was very much discoloured, the left eye half closed from paralysis of the upper eyelid. In spite of all efforts, he was unable to speak a word. Before I arrived they had tried to give him ten globules of S., dry. I immediately ordered S. in dilution, in alternation with A.—at first the second dilution, then the first—one teaspoonful of each remedy to be taken every ten minutes, for half a day. At the same time I applied compresses of A^2 to the head, frequently changed. The next day I added applications of B. E. to the brachial nerves of the paralysed side; also compresses were used above the left eye, to the temples on the same side, and to the region of the heart. With little change, this was continued the whole time. Owing to sleeplessness and strong excitement on the part of the patient, I applied compresses of W. E. to the head, alternately with those of A^2. Later, I again ordered applications of B. E. to the stomach and to the sole of the left foot several times a day. The result of this treatment was most astonishing. In a few days Mr. R. could already move and raise his arm and leg, and pressed my hand vigorously with the affected hand. I do not remember ever having seen such rapid progress in any similar case. After a week, Mr. R. got up and tried to walk a few steps; in a fortnight he walked alone, with the help of a stick, up and down his rooms. Finally, after four weeks, he was so much better that he could come down three flights of stairs, take a walk in the town, and go upstairs to his own rooms again. His eye and mouth had almost regained their normal condition, and his speech was easy and pronunciation clear.

Paralysis. 5. Nervous Paralysis.—Madame P. E., aged 60, had suffered from nervous paralysis for three years. She was completely cured by applications of R. E., and second dilutions of appropriate medicines.

Paralysis.—Mr. F. L., aged 57, had had paralysis in the left upper joints for eight months. The disease was conquered with two applications of R. E.

Phthisis. 1.—P. P., aged 39, suffering for several months from a cough, and attacks of great weakness; his respiration was oppressed; and he had night sweats. Auscultation disclosed proof of *incipient* phthisis. He was cured in four months by S^2 and P^2, in alternation, at first in the second dilutions, then in ordinary doses; and unctions of S^2 alt. C^5 over the chest.

Phthisis. 2.—Mr. N. aged 27, of very delicate constitution, was attacked by tuberculosis on the lungs—palpitation of the heart. Cured by F^2 alt. S^2, and unctions of A^2 on the heart.

Phthisis. 3.—L. F., aged 18, attacked with congestion of the right lung. Cured by P^1, alternately with A., in the second dilutions; and unctions of A^3 on the chest; with applications of B. E.

Phthisis. 4.—B., a boy, aged 12, very weak, thin, pale, constantly fevered; auscultation disclosed a tuberculous cavity under the clavicle. He was cured in four months by alternations, in the second dilution, of P., C., and A.; unctions on the chest of C. and A.; and two globules, dry, every day, of S.

Phthisis. 5.—A girl, aged 13, very weak, spitting blood, night sweats. A sister had died of phthisis at the age of 15. She had C^2, A^2, and P^2, in alternation. After ten days improvement set in, she had no more spitting of blood. The same treatment was continued, and in four months the girl was another creature. Cure was complete.

Phthisis. 6.—A woman, aged 36, with phthisis, well ascertained by experienced observers. The apex of the right lung had been severely affected for five years. She was perfectly cured by alternations in the first dilution of A^3, C., and P.

Phthisis. 7.—A young man, aged 23, given up by five doctors; was completely cured in a few weeks by P. alternately with C. Afterwards S. was continued for some time.

Skin Disease. 1.—Eczema. In a man, aged 50; eczema on the ear; the tube swollen, partly destroyed, suppurating, with extension of the disease around the ear. In three and a half months was completely cured by the first dilution of S., and unctions of S^5. Applications of R. E. to the nape, the temples, and underneath the ear.

Skin. 2.—Eczema and psora over the whole body; had resisted all kinds of treatment for five months. Cured in six weeks by S. internally and externally.

Skin. 3.—Scrofulous eczema around the nostrils, with swelling of the nose and the eyelids. Cured by S. internally and externally.

Skin. 4.—General P., aged 65, had eczema on the hands, which for a year had resisted allopathic treatment. He had rubbed the skin with brushes till blood came. The patient could not sleep on account of intolerable itching. For three months the whole was treated by alternation in dilution of S^5, Ven., and C^5; with unctions and baths of the same remedies.

Skin. 5.—An eczema, of five years' standing, in a lady, due to asthmatic constitution, began at the left ear; a year afterwards it spread to the right ear, then to the scalp, the forehead, temples, the breasts, arms, and thighs. She tried many different treatments, but all were fruitless; the disease only became more intense. In a few months she was completely cured by the following treatment: S. alternately with C. in dilution. Unctions of S^5; compresses of C^5; applications of R. E. At meals, five globules of S., and sometimes of A., in wine. Baths of C^5.

Skin. 6.—An infant, aged 26 months, attacked by skin disease, which showed itself principally by scabs under the left eye, having a diameter of nearly two inches. He had one globule dry of S., night and morning, for about six weeks. During the first three weeks the eruption increased; then it gradually diminished and disappeared.

Lung Disease. 1.—Mr. P., aged 25, retired from military service. The army doctors pronounced the heart, the liver, and the lungs, to be simultaneously affected. He began Electro-homeopathic treatment by alternations of A. and F. in the second dilution; unctions of F^2 to the hypochondria, and of A. to the region of the heart. Six globules dry of S., daily. After three months of this treatment he could scarcely be recognized, so great was the change for the better. He was ultimately cured by P. alternately with C., and applications of W. E.

LUNG DISEASE. 2.—Pleuro-pneumonia. A young girl, aged 12, after suffering for two months from convulsive cough, was attacked by pleuro-pneumonia, with lancinating pains in the left side and shoulder. Temperature, 104°. Expectoration was bloody, and afterwards somewhat like decoction of prunes. In a very short time the pain was subdued, by the use of R. E. In four days the fever was reduced by the second dilution of F., and unctions of F^2 to the hypochondria. Afterwards she had several dry globules of F., and alternations, in the second dilution, of P. and A Improvement was maintained by this treatment, and on the eighth day she left her bed and was entirely restored.

LUNG DISEASE. 3.—Very severe pneumonia in an infant of 8 months, in which pulmonary paralysis seemed impending. After the second spoonful of P. there was an evident return of the receding life; on the next day she was convalescent. Cure was soon attained by P.

LUNG DISEASE. 4.—Pneumonia. N. N., aged 66, after having suffered with peripneumonia three times, was attacked by fever. Temperature 104°; respiration thirty-six a minute. After thirty-six hours, and treatment by alternate use of F., A., and P., with unctions of F^2 to the hypochondria, the thermometer sank to 97°; the characteristic expectoration appeared; percussion and auscultation confirmed the diagnosis of pneumonia, but reduced to a minimum. On the fourth day the patient left his bed, and in six days was cured.

PERITONITIS.—A young woman, aged 26, having suffered from puerperal peritonitis, was cured in a week by constant use of compresses of S^5 and C^{10} and W. E. alternately, and, in the evening, compresses of F^2 to the hypochondria. Internally she had a teaspoonful of the first dilution of C. every quarter of an hour.

ULCER.—A man, aged 70, suffering from a scrofulous ulcer on the left leg, was cured in three months by the internal use of S. and L. alternately, and compresses of L.

PROSTATIC DISEASE. 1.—With catarrh of the bladder, in a man of 71, was cured by S. taken internally, and R. E. applied to the sacrum.

PROSTATIC DISEASE. 2.—Hypertrophy. L. M., aged 56, suffering for three years; in consequence of the hypertrophy he had paralysis of the bladder. He could only be relieved by the use of a catheter. In five months he was cured by the alternate use of S. and A. in the first dilution; baths of L.; unctions of C^5; applications of R. E. to the pubes, the perinæum, the great sympathetic, the solar plexus, and the occiput.

CALCULUS.—Mr. L. O. had had stone for four years. He was cured in a few months by S. internally, and R. E. to the related nerves. The stone was gradually dissolved, and so removed without injury.

RHEUMATISM.—1. Rheumatic gout; rheumatic angina; œdema of the legs. Mr. S., aged 41, of lymphatic temperament, was attacked by œdema of the legs, especially on the right side, with pain and redness near the joints, and great irritation of the surface. These indications pointed to rheumatic gout, and the dryness of the throat, with diffused redness of the fauces and difficult deglutition, pointed to a secondary attack of rheumatic angina.

The disease had resisted allopathic treatment for a year. Then the patient resorted to the Mattei remedies. He was cured in three months by alternation of S. and C., in the first dilution, with the same remedies applied by compresses, and in pulverized form.

RHEUMATISM.—2. Rheumatic gout. A gentleman of lymphatic temperament, who had suffered from rheumatic gout for two years, was cured in one year by the following treatment. One day, twenty globules of S., dry; that is, one every half hour. The next day A., taken in the same manner. Alternate applications externally of R. E. and W. E. Baths of L. alternately with W. E.

RHEUMATISM. 3.—Father Falrice, aged 30, living at Bologna, suffered extremely from chronic rheumatism, owing to suppressed perspiration. The rheumatism was subdued by the internal use of S., and alternate applications of R. E. and Y. E.

RHEUMATISM. 4.—A lady, aged 40, suffering from rheumatism, with chronic granular inflammation of the tonsils, leucorrhœa and pains in the renal regions; was cured in a few months by L., in dilution. Gargles of A^2; unctions of C^5; baths of L.

RICKETS.—A son of Mr. K., aged 6, suffered from rickets. The knees were distorted, also the feet, the arms, and the chest. He was thin, pale, unhealthy looking, weak, a little model of decrepitude. He was radically cured in eight months by the first dilution of S.; unctions and baths of S. alternately with C^5. Application of R. E., alternately with Y., E. to all the nerve centres.

SCROFULA. 1.—Miss A., aged 24, had had scrofulous ulcers on both feet for three years; declared incurable. She was cured in two months with complete cicatrization, by internal use of Ven. and S^5 alternately.

SCROFULA. 2.—The Marquis of M. D., aged 62. had suffered from scrofulous ulceration of the left nostril for many years. The disease had resisted all treatment, even C^5 and S^5, internally and externally. They were changed for A^2, alternately with Ven., in the second dilution, and pulverized Ven. applied externally. After three weeks a notable amelioration was produced, and the ulceration assumed an entirely different character. After three months' treatment the cure was complete.

SCROFULA. 3.—The Rev. Antoine Bellerini, a Jesuit Father, professor at the College Romain, aged 65, suffering from constitutional and advanced scrofula, was completely cured in seven months by A. and S., used internally.

SCROFULA. 1.—A child, aged 3; the eyes had not been open for three months, the nose covered with scabs, also he could not urinate. The ophthalmic surgeons and the general physicians tried in vain to cure him. He was then put under Mattei treatment, and in four months was cured by the following treatment. First dilutions of S. and A. alternately. Eye water and lotions of A^3, 15 globules in two-thirds of a tumblerful of water.

DEAFNESS.—H., aged 24, had violent headaches, running from the ears, complete deafness of one ear, for six months. Cured in three weeks by R. E., S. in dilution, and injections of S.

SCIATICA. 1.—T. R., aged 44, had suffered from sciatica for five months. Cured in twenty-five days by S., first dilution, applications externally of R. B. alternately with F. to the sciatic nerve.

SCIATICA. 2.—Acute sciatica. P. B., aged 40; cured in three days by S. in dilution. Applications of W. E. Baths of C^5.

SCIATICA. 3.—Chronic sciatica. S. G., aged 41, had suffered from sciatica for three years. Cured by a few applications of R. E. without internal treatment.

SCIATICA. 4.—J. B., suffering from sciatica, which was declared to be incurable by allopathic methods; was cured in three weeks by S., and applications alternately of R. E. and Y. E.

SCIATICA. 5.—With biliary calculi (gall stones). Mrs. N. V., aged 42; cured by first dilution of F., baths of S. and C. alternately; applications of R. E. alternately with Y. E. to the sciatic nerve, and compresses of W. E. to the sciatic nerve; and compresses of W. E. to the solar plexus, to the kidney region, and the sympathetic.

SYPHILIS. 1.—Mr. J. C., aged 59, with chancrous ulcers, was completely cured by Ven. internally and externally, and baths of the same remedy.

SYPHILIS. 2.—Mr. P. P., aged 38, had suffered from syphilis for ten years; all treatment had failed. In one month he was perfectly cured by the internal use of Ven.

SYPHILIS. 3.—Condylomata. Mr. M. A., aged 32, was cured in a short time by the internal use of A.

SYPHILIS. 4.—*Adenitis.* Mr. P. D., aged 40, suffering from ulcerated state of the glands of the groin; a very serious state on account of the depth of the local disease, the character of the discharge, and the unhealthy condition of the borders of the ulcers. By the use of A. internally, and compresses of the same, he was in two months entirely cured.

SYPHILIS. 5.—Ulcers. Mr. P., aged 19, had phagedemic ulcers; cured in a fortnight by A. alternately with Ven., internally and externally.

SYPHILIS. 6.—Chronic blennorrhagia. P. S., aged 36, had indolent ulcers and chronic blennorrhagia. He began treatment on February 21, and was completely cured, on April 5, by Ven. and S. alternately and internally.

SYPHILIS. 7.—T. L., aged 17, suffered from discharge and an abscess on the left groin for several months. Complete cure was effected by Ven. internally, and baths of C5.

SYPHILIS. 8.—Mr. B. C., aged 51, had constitutional pains and ulcers on the palate. In two months he was completely cured by Ven. internally, and internal applications of W. E. alternately with B. E.

SYPHILIS. 9.—T. P., aged 26, suffered from venereal ulcerations, and was pronounced incurable by Professor Gamberini, after eight years' treatment of different kinds. In only three weeks he was cured by Ven., alternately with C^5 in dilution. Alternate compresses of C^4 and Ven. Internal treatment was continued for some months.

SYPHILIS. 10.—A man, aged 28, had had boils for five months. Was cured in four weeks by the following treatment. Ven. internally, lotions and unctions of Ven. externally. After ten days the treatment was changed to S^2. externally, unctions of S., baths of S. (50 globules).

SYPHILIS. 11.—L. G., aged 22, had inguinal adenitis (glandular inflammation) with deep ulcerations locally. He was cured in a fortnight by Ven. internally and externally.

SYPHILIS. 12.—Blepharitis. A man, aged 62, gradually lost his sight. Inflammation had destroyed the eyes, which were bathed in thick suppuration, resembling two gaping wounds. He was cured in four months by S. and Ven. used internally; lotions to the eyes, and compresses of C^5 and S^5.

HEAD CASES.

HEADACHE. 1.—Daily Cephalalgia. Mrs. C., aged 32, several years ago had intermittent fever, with daily headache, which subsequently developed into migraine—sometimes on the right, sometimes on the left side. She was cured in two months by F., in the second dilution, and compresses of F^2 to the hypochondria.

HEADACHE. 2.—Mr. K., aged 16, had suffered from headache for three years, hindering study; and pronounced incurable. He was cured by the use of W. E.

HEADACHE. 3.—Periodical. G. P., aged 35; cured by A. alternately with A^3. in dilution.

HEADACHE. 4.—Mrs. B. M., aged 47, had been afflicted with periodical nervous headache for several months. All the usual remedies had been tried in vain. She was cured by S. in dilution, baths of L., and applications of W. E. to the head.

HEADACHE. 5.—A. P., aged 29, had suffered for two years from violent headaches, with vertigo, returning every month, and lasting from eight to twelve days. He could neither read nor walk, and was obliged to remain shut up in his darkened chamber. He was radically cured by the first dilution of A., compresses of B. E. to the heart, of B. E. to the head, and of F^2 to the hypochondria.

TETANUS.—D. M. had tetanus in the right arm, consequent upon an injury to the hand. The tetanus was cured by Y. E. alone, applied to the occiput. The injury was cured by compresses of A.

COUGH. 1.—Miss M., aged 18, had suffered for six months from cough, with expectoration of a suspicious character, and general emaciation. She had oppressed breathing on going upstairs. She was cured in five weeks by P. in dilution.

COUGH. 2.—Mr. M. O., aged 75, suffered from a very violent cough, preventing sleep at night; he was much weakened. P^3, which was thought applicable, had no effect, and it was changed the next day to P^4. In two days the cough, which had lasted a long time, disappeared entirely, and the old man felt remarkably well.

COUGH. 3.—A child, aged 6, retained a cough from inflammation of the lungs which he had had some months previously; he had also tubercles at the top of the right lung. He was cured radically by S. alternately with P. in the second dilution, and inhalations of P^2.

TIC-DOLOREUX.—P. T. has suffered from tic-doloreux and chronic neuralgia for twenty years. By the use of S. internally, and compresses of the same, and applications of R. E., he was completely cured.

ECZEMATOUS ERUPTION. 1.—A young girl, aged 8, of mixed temperament. Eczema covered her head with sores, and there was an ulcer on the lower right eyelid. This disease returned every spring. She had been always treated by a regular doctor, but her disease had been only relieved, not cured. She was put under the Mattei treatment, and in six weeks was cured by the internal use of S. For two years the disease has not returned.

ECZEMA. 2.—A woman, aged 22, had already been treated for eczema without success. She was cured in five weeks by alternate use of S. and A., with unctions of C^5.

TUMOUR.—A man, aged 22, of angioitic temperament, had an internal abdominal tumour, with swelling and tumefaction of the body from the chest to the thighs, which were very hard and discoloured. The doctors had given him up as incurable;

and he had not, so they said, more than a few days to live. In three months he was perfectly cured by the use of A., C^5, and S., in alternation, and in the second dilutions; with 3 globules of S. at meal-times; compresses and unctions of C. and L. alternately.

Worms.

Worms.—The vermifugo medicines, taken dry, produce wonderful effects. Five globules cut short nervous attacks, whether due to worms or not; also certain painful periodical disorders of the stomach; such is its remarkable action on the nervous system. Here we had clear evidence of the electric action of the remedy, and that Electro-Homœopathy attacks the causes of disease, seeing that a remedy against worms has such extraordinary nervine effects; and that, on the other hand, worms themselves produce profound changes in the nervous system.

In worm cases the effect of Vermifugo in massive doses and in dilution is not the same, while the dilution brings away the worms in fragments, accompanied by glairy mucus, and few at a time; when taken dry they bring away the worms, if not living, yet almost entire.

Another property of the Vermifugos is that, with children suffering from bronchial disease with accumulation of phlegm, as in whooping-cough, 4 or 5 globules, taken dry, cause a large quantity of glairy mucus to pass by the evacuations, and thus prevent the frequent return of paroxysms of cough.

A woman of 28, suffering from tænia, which had resisted the action of Rousso, after suffering convulsions at intervals for seven years, was cured by very small doses of Ver.

Worms. 2.—A. P., a little girl, aged 7, presented all the indications of being afflicted with worms. After eleven days' use of Ver. she was seized by a terrible convulsion, which the doctors called epilepsy. However, she passed a quantity of lumbrici, all dead, and from that time suffered no longer from the disorder which had before afflicted her.

Varicose Veins.—Varicose ulcers. A. Vergignani, aged 48, of Bologna, had been troubled with varicose ulcers on the right leg for four years. He was cured in three months by the internal use of A. The external treatment evidently accelerated cure.

Sight. 1.—*Ophthalmia.* Mr. T. A., aged 45, had chronic granular ophthalmia. He was treated for some time without result at the Ophthalmic Ward, at Bologna. He was cured in seven weeks by S. internally, and applications externally of W. E.

Sight. 2.—*Incipient Amaurosis.* Mr. F. H., aged 32, suffered from incipient amaurosis, and permanent contraction of the left pupil. It was supposed to have arisen from exhalations of carbonic acid gas. By the use of R. E. improvement set in at once; cured by A. internally, and (compresses) externally. He was cured in a month.

Sight. 3.—*Granular Ophthalmia.* C. G., aged 23, suffering from granular inflammation; was cured in six months by A. given internally, and the external application of W. E.

Sight. 4.—*Ophthalmia.* E. V., aged 6, was tormented with granular ophthalmia, and was cured in a month by S. internally and externally.

Sight. 5.—*Chronic Ophthalmia.* T. C., on March 21st, began treatment for chronic ophthalmia resulting from syphilis. Also he had a seton in his back. On April 10th, he left the hospital perfectly cured, having been treated by A. and Ver. in alternation.

Sight. 6.—*Granular Ophthalmia.* T. F., aged 5. Suffering from granular ophthalmia. For three months he was treated by allopathy without success. In seven weeks he was cured by S. in dilution, and applications of W. E. to the occiput and over the eyes.

Sight. 7.—*Staphyloma.* R. M., aged 77, had staphyloma in the left eye. Several physicians and professors declared the disease incurable. He was, however, cured in eight months by S. taken internally, and used externally.

INDEX.

UNWIN BROTHERS, THE GRESHAM PRESS, CHILWORTH AND LONDON.